Epidemiological
Psychiatry

Publication Number 864

AMERICAN LECTURE SERIES®

A Monograph in

The BANNERSTONE DIVISION *of*
AMERICAN LECTURES IN LIVING CHEMISTRY

Edited by

I. NEWTON KUGELMASS, M.D., Ph.D., Sc.D.
Consultant to the Departments of Health and Hospitals
New York City

Epidemiological Psychiatry

By

BRIAN COOPER, M.D., M.R.C. Psych., D.P.M.

Senior Lecturer, Institute of Psychiatry
University of London
Honorary Consultant, Bethlem Royal and Maudsley Hospitals
London, England

and

H. G. MORGAN, M.A., M.B., M.R.C.P.,
M.R.C. Psych., D.P.M.

Senior Lecturer in Mental Health
University of Bristol
Honorary Consultant, United Bristol Hospital and
Southwestern Regional Hospital Board, England.

With a Foreword by

MICHAEL SHEPHERD

Professor of Epidemiological Psychiatry
University of London

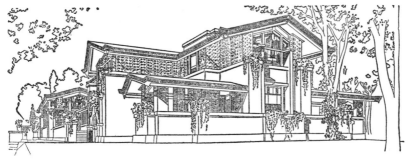

CHARLES C THOMAS · PUBLISHER
Springfield · Illinois · U.S.A.

Published and Distributed Throughout the World by
CHARLES C THOMAS • PUBLISHER
BANNERSTONE HOUSE
301-327 East Lawrence Avenue, Springfield, Illinois, U.S.A.

© *1973, by* CHARLES C THOMAS • PUBLISHER

ISBN 0-398-02581-9

Library of Congress Catalog Card Number: 72-869982

With THOMAS BOOKS *careful attention is given to all details of manufacturing and design. It is the Publisher's desire to present books that are satisfactory as to their physical qualities and artistic possibilities and appropriate for their particular use.* THOMAS BOOKS *will be true to those laws of quality that assure a good name and good will.*

Printed in the United States of America
N-10

EDITOR'S FOREWORD

OUR LIVING CHEMISTRY SERIES was conceived by Editor and Publisher to advance the newer knowledge of chemical medicine in the cause of clinical practice. The interdependence of chemistry and medicine is so great that physicians are turning to chemistry, and chemists to medicine in order to understand the underlying basis of life processes in health and disease. Once chemical truths, proofs and convictions become foundations for clinical phenomena, key hybrid investigators clarify the bewildering panorama of biochemical progress for application in everyday practice, stimulation of experimental research, and extension of postgraduate instruction. Each of our monographs thus unravels the chemical mechanisms and clinical management of many diseases that have remained relatively static in the minds of medical men for three thousand years. Our new Series is charged with the *nisus élan* of chemical wisdom, supreme in choice of international authors, optimal in standards of chemical scholarship, provocative in imagination for experimental research, comprehensive in discussion of scientific medicine, and authoritative in chemical perspective of human disorders.

Dr. Cooper of London and Dr. Morgan of Bristol, extend their activities beyond the traditional clinical focus on individual patients to the deep-seated concern for communitywide problems of mental health and mental illness. On the basis of considerable experience in England they find a direct correlation between poverty and style of life and prevalence of mental illnesses, but the major mental disorders—schizophrenia and manic-depressive psychoses—occur in all known families of man in not too highly dissimilar rates. The role of social forces in causing mental illness has been recognized for centuries; hence epidemiology takes all morbidity for its province—mental, physical and emotional illnesses—as a collective science. Future progress in psychiatry will depend largely on effective integration of clinical, experimental and epidemiological studies en masse. It will require the heterodoxy of the fully informed scholar who rebels against orthodoxy within himself and within his own camp.

The main value of psychiatric epidemiology is in identifying the determinants of mental illness or deviant behavior growing out of the interaction between man and his environment in ensuring the effective deployment of services available for treatment and prevention. The epidemiologist examines the prevalence and relates the data on the amount of morbidity to personal, social, geographical, or temporal factors. The survey must be carried out in the setting in which people naturally exist and the people must be representative of the population studied. After each person has been screened for the conditions in question, the number identifiable as ill, disturbed, or maladjusted can then be determined. The psychoses and subnormalities can be so studied fairly well but the neuroses, character anomalies, and psychopathic states present great difficulties. Epidemiological psychiatry may be narrowly conceived as getting at problems in an early stage or widely conceived as the psychiatric contribution to a new venture of constructing new cultural forms, from within which individuals of hitherto nonexisting types of strength and new vulnerabilities as well, will emerge to put into practice our rapidly developing body of insights about human nature.

The tasks of the future are infinitely more difficult and call for a much higher degree of cooperation between a larger variety of interested workers in diverse disciplines. The enemies of our health are not in the major diseases due to microorganisms; in many cases they are not even killing diseases, but they cause an immense amount of invalidity. To suppress them, we require accurate knowledge and observation and studies of all the environmental factors. The field is wide, the horizon is not in sight, the tasks are tempting and of tremendous interest worldwide. The investigation of the factors which make for mutual health are more fascinating and infinitely more useful than the cure of established disease. The prospect before psychiatric epidemiologists was never brighter. As for the future, the task is not to foresee, but to enable it.

Most people have some degree of mental illness at some time, And many have a degree of mental illness most of the time.

I. NEWTON KUGELMASS, M.D., Ph.D., Sc.D., *Editor*

FOREWORD

Familia sic putant omnes quae jam factor, nec de salebris cogitant, ubi via strata (When a thing has once been done, people think it easy; when the road is made, they forget how rough the way used to be).

This Latin dictum applies well to the construction of a first textbook which represents a landmark in the evolution of any medical or scientific field of study. The author must shoulder the responsibility not only of marshalling his material and demarcating its boundaries but also of deciding the form in which it is to be presented. The task is relatively straightforward when new facts or technical achievements are to be presented in a well-established framework, as with such subjects as cytogenetics or neuroendocrinology. It is more complex when concepts and methods associated with other disciplines have to be both incorporated and given a different perspective, as in the case of psychopharmacology or medical sociology.

What has come to be known as epidemiological psychiatry clearly falls into this second category. Its roots are manifold, and are entangled with those of topics as diverse as biostatistics, sociology, psychology, public health administration, genetics, demography, and clinical psychiatry. Its emergence as an independent, synthetic discipline in its own right is a matter of some historical interest which Doctors Cooper and Morgan outline clearly in their first chapter. The bulk of their book is then devoted to three aims which, in their own words are "to identify the outstanding problems of method, to define the scope of epidemiology in the study of mental disorders, and to begin to discern the probable directions of future research."

They have succeeded admirably in achieving all these objectives. In so doing they have brought together a mass of information which will be of interest to public health workers, clinicians

ix

and experimentalists concerned with the various forms of mental disorder. Equally important, they have provided a compact, lucid and authoritative review which can be employed for educational purposes by teachers and pupils alike. With the increasing awareness of the significance of epidemiological psychiatry their book appears at an opportune time and merits a warm welcome.

MICHAEL SHEPHERD, D.M., F.R.C.P.,
F.R.C.Psych., D.P.M., F.A.P.H.A.
Professor of Epidemiological Psychiatry,
Institute of Psychiatry,
University of London

INTRODUCTION

E<small>PIDEMIOLOGY HAS BEEN DEFINED</small> as "the study of the distribution of disease in time and space, and of the factors that influence this distribution" (280). Hence, it shares much common ground with *medical ecology*, which is the study of disease in relation to man's environment, of the conditions under which any given disease tends to occur and to flourish. In this sense, epidemiology and medical ecology both derive from that tradition of study of the "natural history" of disease which can be traced back to Thomas Sydenham and, indeed, to Hippocrates (179).

In the past, the term epidemiology was equated with the study of *epidemics,* which in turn were defined as large outbreaks of acute, infectious disease. This usage is now regarded as unduly restrictive, on two counts. In the first place, it is recognized that the prevalence of any disease, including those which are not directly communicable, may wax and wane: thus, the recent massive increases in Western society of bronchial carcinoma and of ischaemic heart disease can justifiably be called epidemics. Secondly, the same methods which in the nineteenth century were applied so effectively to the problems of infectious fevers now play an important part in the study of such "crowd diseases" as cancer, coronary artery disease, chronic bronchitis, nutritional disorders, congenital defects and even road traffic accidents. In short, epidemiology as the basic science of public health today takes all morbidity for its province. The purpose of this book is to review the scope and methods of epidemiology in the study of mental disorders.

That mental illness and defect represent major public health problems can scarcely be questioned while these conditions account for nearly half of all hospital beds, and rank high among the causes of chronic disablement. It is in these terms that they have come to be seen as legitimate targets for epidemiological research. A decade ago, this change of viewpoint was clearly enunciated in a report of the World Health Organization:

> The problems of studying personal susceptibility and the modifying effects of the environment or habit on the risks of attack were essentially similar in the communicable diseases and in other kinds of human illness. Consequently, the methods which had been used so successfully in uncovering the origin and mode of spread of diseases associated with microbial infection came to be increasingly applied to the study of mental disorders, and the use of the term "epidemiology" to imply the study of their distribution and behaviour in differing conditions of life in human communities became widely accepted (483).

The ensuing convergence of two professional disciplines has been accompanied by some misgiving on both sides. Epidemiologists' doubts have centred on the difficulties of definition and case-detection which seem inseparable from the study of mental disorders in the community. Some have implied that under these conditions the attempt to use epidemiological methods may be premature, an argument which, though losing force with the passage of time, cannot yet be dismissed. A large part of the book is taken up by a consideration of these and related problems of method, and of the extent to which they have been, or can be, overcome.

The sceptical attitude of some psychiatrists relates to a more fundamental issue, namely, how far population studies can ever throw light on the complexities of individual human psychology. This question goes far beyond the scope of the present volume, although some of the work here reviewed is undoubtedly relevant to the argument. It may be as well, however, to make two basic points at the outset. First, although epidemiology deals with populations, its findings depend ultimately on the diagnosis and clinical assessment of individuals. If measures based on these judgments are not deemed valid for study of the mass aspects of mental disorder, it is hard to see how they can be valid for clinical and experimental research in the same field. In other words, the epidemiological approach stands or falls by the applicability of scientific method as a whole.

Secondly, it must be emphasized that the use of survey techniques does not require allegiance to any school of psychiatry.

Admittedly, population studies of mental disorder have tended in the past to draw their inspiration largely from genetic theories; today, however, they are equally likely to derive from environmental or psychodynamic hypotheses. Whether or not the disease model in its traditional sense is basic to epidemiological psychiatry must be considered a semantic question. As Mechanic (321) has pointed out, the epidemiologist's methods are by no means unique, but are shared with sociologists, social psychologists and other non-medical workers who engage in survey research. In the investigation of such forms of social deviance as alcoholism, drug addiction and delinquency, the boundary between medical and sociological research is extremely ill defined; nor can it be demarcated by reference to underlying pathological processes. Epidemiology as a *collective* science must constantly adapt itself to changing concepts of health and morbidity.

The distinctive feature of epidemiology as a mode of enquiry is its concern with geographically defined populations. This concern may be expressed either in estimating the prevalence of disease in a population, or in studying how disease incidence varies with the strength of environmental factors. The two methods are sometimes referred to as *descriptive* and *analytical* epidemiology respectively, though the distinction is far from clear-cut.

A number of ways of categorizing epidemiological research have been employed in reviews of the subject. The outstanding account by Morris (331) of the 'uses' of epidemiology, though criticized on theoretical grounds (449), has undoubtedly had a wide influence. Morris' principal categories were community diagnosis, completion of the clinical picture of disease, delineation of new syndromes, computation of individual morbid risk, charting of historical trends, evaluation of health services in action, and identification of causal factors: all of these find application in psychiatry (422, 172), although there is wide overlap between the categories. Some authors have used a different approach, based on types of research strategy (379, 389); others again have classified published studies according to the factors—genetic, somatic, psychosocial, etc.—on which the research has focussed (284). Finally, a simple threefold typology has been employed

(79) which depends on whether the principal research aim has to do with the planning of medical services, with clinical aspects of disease, or with the scientific investigation of aetiology. This system has the advantage of being readily comprehensible to workers in other fields, and of emphasizing the relevance of epidemiology to their own spheres of activity; for this reason, it has been incorporated into the framework of the present volume.

The book's contents have been arranged as far as possible according to a logical sequence. Chapter 1 provides a brief historical sketch of the growth of epidemiology as a science, and of its early applications in psychiatry. Chapter 2 comprises a general introduction to the principles and methods of epidemiology, with special reference to the study of mental disorders. The next three chapters outline the scope of epidemiology in modern psychiatry: Chapter 3 deals with the planning of mental health services, Chapter 4 with the enlargement of clinical perspectives, and Chapter 5 with the search for causal factors. Chapter 6 attempts, however inadequately, to review current progress in this subspecialty and to show how it is related to advances in a number of research fields. The sequence gives rise to one discontinuity, in that questions of concept and method raised in Chapter 2 have to be taken up again in Chapter 6. Some readers may prefer, therefore, to take these two chapters in conjunction, in the same way that Chapters 3, 4 and 5 may be read as a whole.

This arrangement of the material serves to present a selective, and to some extent personal, view of epidemiological psychiatry which has evolved over a number of years, largely as a result of collaboration and discussion with colleagues at the Institute of Psychiatry and elsewhere. In particular, some of the ideas expressed here have already been set out in a number of review articles, written by one of the authors with Professor Michael Shepherd (78, 79, 422) . No attempt has been made to cover epidemiological research on any of the major psychiatric categories, nor to review the literature on such broad themes as the relationship of psychiatric morbidity to age, sex, marital status or social class. The references in the text have been selected to illustrate particular points, and are not intended to be comprehensive; for convenience, they have been largely restricted to English-language publications. Lack of space has permitted only cursory mention of work in such closely related areas of research as population genetics and medical statistics. In many instances, reference has been made to key review articles which provide extensive bibliographies, and the reader should consult these for further information.

The principal theme of this book is that future progress in psychiatric research will depend largely on the successful integration of clinical, experimental and epidemiological programmes; its basic underlying premise is that population studies of mental disorder should be undertaken by, or with the full support of, those responsible for its treatment and management. If they succeed in communicating these ideas to even a small proportion of professional workers in the mental health field, the authors will have achieved their objective.

CONTENTS

Epidemiological
Psychiatry

Chapter One

HISTORICAL BACKGROUND

T HAT SOME FORMS of mental disorder can behave, in their mass aspects, like the major communicable diseases is a fact repeatedly attested to over the centuries. Large-scale outbreaks of bizarre, irrational behaviour have occurred periodically in all societies throughout history, their appearance often coinciding with periods of severe social disruption (78). In his treatise on the epidemics of the Middle Ages, Hecker (190) treats such disorders as dancing mania, tarantism and flagellation in the same terms as the contagious diseases of the time, invoking "sympathy" or "imitation" as the agent of transmission. Graphic descriptions of these phenomena abound, yet only in recent times has any kind of mental disorder begun to be studied by the methods of scientific epidemiology.

It is no accident that these methods were first established in the field of acute infectious disease. Here, problems of definition and case-detection were relatively straightforward, while the occurrence of epidemics with manifest person-to-person spread emphasized the need for preventive measures, based on a knowledge of the mode of transmission of each disease. Moreover, mass outbreaks of plague, cholera and typhus appeared to correspond to the simplest of epidemiological models: that in which a single pathogen acts as the necessary and sufficient cause of disease, while variations in susceptibility are of minor importance. In these circumstances, the epidemiologist can afford to neglect the first factor in the triad of Host, Agent and Environment, and to concentrate on the nature of the pathogenic agent, its mode of spread and the climatic and other environmental conditions which favour its dissemination. No better example can be given of this type of investigation than the classic studies of John Snow on the London cholera outbreaks of the mid-nineteenth century (71).

3

JOHN SNOW ON CHOLERA

Snow's work is outstanding alike for the meticulous care of his observation and recording, the essentially modern nature of his hypothetico-deductive approach and, finally, the stroke of genius by which he took advantage of the opportunity of a natural experiment to put his beliefs to the test.

In his preliminary assessment of what at the time was a major scourge, Snow seized upon three features of cholera which appeared to him to hold the key to its mode of spread. First, the disease began with alimentary tract symptoms. Secondly, people who had shared the same room with a fatal case did not necessarily contract cholera. For example, although at the Tooting Institution for pauper children and lunatics the death rate in one cholera epidemic rose as high as 140 per 1,000 inmates, the staff, or "keepers" as they were known, suffered remarkably little. Finally, cholera outbreaks occurred in a pattern of widely dispersed multiple foci, rather than in the type of localized spread one would expect from direct person-to-person contagion.

Snow concluded that the pathogenic agent, the "materies morbi" of cholera, whose nature was quite unknown, was most probably conveyed by oral intake, the likeliest culprit being contaminated drinking water. He noted many examples of an apparent relationship between the spread of disease and the type of local water supply. In the London suburb of Ilford in 1849, for example, he found that all the houses in one row had been affected, with a single exception where the inhabitants had refused to consume the local water because of its offensive nature. Again, he noted:

> In Albion Terrace, Wandsworth Road, there was an extraordinary mortality from cholera in 1849 which was the more striking as there were no other cases at the time in the immediate neighbourhood: the houses opposite to, behind and in the same line, at each end of those in which the disease prevailed, having been free from it. The row of houses in which the cholera prevailed to an extent probably at that time unprecedented in this country constituted the genteel suburban dwelling of a number of professional and trades people and are most of them detached a few feet from each other. They were supplied

with water on the same plan. In this instance the water got contaminated by the contents of the house drains and cesspools. The cholera extended to nearly all the houses in which the water was thus tainted, and to no others.

In the same year, 1849, occurred what Snow called "the most terrible outbreak" in the Broad Street and Golden Square area of central London. Within an area of a few city blocks there were more than five hundred fatal cases of cholera in ten days, a mortality exceeding even that of the plague two centuries earlier. Suspecting contamination of the water supplied by the Broad Street pump, Snow obtained from the General Register Office a list of cholera deaths in the area and located the houses in which they occurred; since all were in closer proximity to Broad Street than to any other source of water, it seemed likely that their inhabitants had used the suspected pump. By enquiring at each of the affected houses, he was able to confirm that there had been no outbreak or increase in cholera in that part of London except among persons who had drawn water from the Broad Street pump.

Snow was well aware of the deficiencies in his data at this stage; he noted that many local inhabitants had fled the area when the outbreak occurred, some possibly to die elsewhere; moreover, those who died in the local workhouse did not have their home addresses recorded, and some fatal cases in hospital had also come from unknown addresses. Nevertheless, after careful assessment, he decided that these factors were unlikely to have been responsible for any serious bias in his findings.

As a result of this investigation, Snow felt on sufficiently firm ground to have the handle of the Broad Street pump removed, so as to prevent people from using the contaminated water. The local epidemic was already on the wane, so that removal of the pump handle was probably only a minor factor in the subsequent rapid fall in infection. Nonetheless, his action acquired a symbolic significance which has made it a landmark in the history of epidemiology.

At that time, drinking water was supplied to London south of the River Thames by two commercial firms, the Southwark and

Vauxhall Company and the Lambeth Company; both obtained their water from the river at Battersea where it was heavily contaminated with sewage. The incidence of cholera in areas supplied by these companies was found to be greater than anywhere else in London. Using statistics on cholera compiled by Farr and death-rates for each area of London published by the General Register Office, Snow calculated that in 1849 there was a cholera mortality of one in sixty amongst consumers of water from each of the two companies. Soon afterwards, the Lambeth Company moved its works further up the river to an area free from sewage pollution. Snow argued that if contaminated drinking water was an important factor in cholera spread, the incidence of the disease in areas supplied by the Lambeth Company should decrease with the improvement in the purity of its water supply. When the next epidemic occurred in 1853, he was able to show that this change did in fact occur. His findings are summarized in Table I.

TABLE I
DISTRICT MORTALITY FROM CHOLERA BY SOURCE OF WATER
SUPPLY: SOUTH LONDON, 1853

Water Supply	*No. of Subdistricts*	*Population in 1851*	*Deaths by Cholera in Each 100,000 Living in Subdistrict*
Southwark & Vauxhall	12	167,654	114
Both Companies	16	301,149	60
Lambeth Company	3	14,632	—

Source: Adapted from Snow on Cholera (71).

During the cholera epidemic of the following year, 1854, Snow conceived and carried out his crucial experiment. In order to confirm his hypothesis, he needed to compare the incidence of cholera in relation to each water supply in an area where the two companies were directly competing. In this situation, all other variables such as geographical area, social class and overcrowding would be eliminated as in a controlled trial. The theoretical basis is best described in Snow's own words:

> In the sub-districts where both companies supply water, the mixing of the supply is of the most intimate kind. The pipes of each company

go down all the streets and into nearly all the courts and alleys. A few houses are supplied by one company and a few by the other, according to the decision of the owners at the time when the companies were in active competition. In many cases a single house is supplied by a different company from that on either side. Each company supplies both rich and poor, both large and small houses; there is no difference either in the conditions or occupations of the persons receiving the water of the different companies.

Having first obtained from the General Register Office the addresses of fatal cholera cases in the area to be studied, Snow then set out with a single assistant, John Whiting, to visit all the houses where fatalities had occurred. By this personal enquiry the source of the water supply was ascertained for every house: a prodigious task. In those instances where the source of water to a household could not be ascertained, he carried out a chloride test which distinguished the tidal water of the Southwark and Vauxhall Company from that drawn by their competitor from the higher reaches of the Thames. The results of his enquiry are shown in Table II.

TABLE II
HOUSEHOLD MORTALITY FROM CHOLERA BY SOURCE OF WATER
SUPPLY: SOUTH LONDON, 1854

Water Supply	Total Number of Houses Supplied	Deaths From Cholera in Districts Investigated	Death rate in Each 10,000 Houses Supplied
Southwark & Vauxhall	40,046	1,263	315
Lambeth Co.	26,107	98	37
Rest of London	256,423	1,422	59

Source: Adapted from Snow on Cholera (71).

It can be seen that the mortality in houses supplied by the Southwark and Vauxhall Company was eight or nine times as great as in those supplied by the Lambeth Company. Indeed, customers of the latter suffered less from cholera than the rest of London, despite the fact that they were living in the worst affected area of the city.

At the time of this investigation, Snow was unable to calculate accurate cholera mortality rates for each water-supply within his defined area, because he knew only the total number of houses supplied by each water company in London. It was not until 1856 that he obtained statistics to show that the cholera mortality amongst Southwark and Vauxhall consumers as a whole was six times that among consumers of the Lambeth Company. Nevertheless, the case he had presented for a water-borne spread of cholera was already overwhelming.

Snow's work on cholera was the prototype for those studies of the transmission of infectious disease which were to remain the chief preoccupation of epidemiologists for the next half-century and more. All his evidence was circumstantial, resting on statistical observations and relationships; yet he was able, thirty years before Koch discovered the cholera vibrio, to show how the disease was spread and how it might be prevented. In the words of Bradford Hill: "For almost 100 years we have been free in this country from epidemic cholera, and it is a freedom which basically we owe to the logical thinking, acute observation and simple sums of John Snow" (198).

With the development of bacterial techniques and immunology, the need for painstaking studies of the distribution and mode of spread of infectious disease became less apparent, and the focus of interest shifted to the laboratory. Not all epidemic diseases, however, yielded to bacteriological investigation. In the nutritional deficiencies, for example, where specific causal agents operate as surely as in the infectious fevers, the search for pathogenic organisms was in vain. One such condition, pellagra, was thought to be a contagious disease until its true cause was revealed by one of the most outstanding of all epidemiological enquiries, and one of the first to have direct implications for psychiatry.

GOLDBERGER ON PELLAGRA

Pellagra is a disease with important psychiatric aspects, being responsible for a variety of neurasthenic symptoms and, in a small minority of cases, for a well-defined psychosis. In 1914, when Joseph Goldberger of the United States Public Health Service was assigned to the problem, there was alarm at the progressive increase in this condition. Expert opinion at that time mostly favoured an infectious aetiology; indeed, the Thompson-McFadden Commission had recently suggested that pellagra was a specific communicable disease (429, 430). Their conclusion was based on an observed association of new with pre-existing cases, an apparent relationship with poor sanitation, and the results of a house-to-house survey of more than 5,000 people in areas of endemic pellagra, which revealed no link with faulty diet.

Within a few months of starting work, Goldberger had arrived at a diametrically opposed viewpoint, namely, that the cause was entirely dietary (150, 151). Like John Snow before him, Goldberger arrived at his central hypothesis by a process of inductive reasoning from a handful of observations which he held to be of prime significance. To begin with, in institutions where pellagra was rife no cases were reported among nurses or attendants. Moreover, fresh cases occurred among patients who had been inmates continuously for many years, and who had had no contact with the outside world. These facts spoke strongly against an infective origin. Secondly, the highest prevalence of pellagra was to be found in rural areas, whose inhabitants were known to have less varied and nourishing diets than those of town dwellers. Finally, the known association between pellagra and poverty also suggested the likelihood of a dietary cause.

One of Goldberger's earliest studies was carried out at an orphanage in Jackson, Mississippi. Here, in the year 1914, no fewer than 68 children, or nearly one third of the residents, suffered from pellagra. A very high incidence was found among those aged six to twelve years, a finding whose significance Goldberger was quick to grasp:

> Inasmuch as all live under identical environmental conditions, the remarkable exemption of the group of younger and that of the older children is no more comprehensible on the basis of an infection than is the absolute immunity of the asylum employees (151).

The explanation, he believed, lay in the fact that whereas the younger children were given a daily ration of fresh milk, and those over twelve years received supplementary food as farmworkers, the children of between six and twelve years subsisted on the basic orphanage diet.

Goldberger, unlike Snow, was able to confirm his hypothesis by proceeding to experimental research. In a series of investigations, he and his associates demonstrated how pellagra could be prevented by improving institutional diets (154) and how, on the other hand, dietary restriction could lead to its appearance (155). They were able to prevent new cases in two orphanages, which for years had been endemic foci of pellagra, by increasing the supply of fresh animal and leguminous foods while other factors remained constant. At the Georgia State Sanatorium, where similar results were obtained, nearly half of a group of 32 control patients showed recurrence of pellagra during a one-year survey period. When the experimental group returned to the ordinary institutional diet, their incidence of pellagra increased sharply, only to fall again when the diet was improved once more (153). These results showed conclusively that pellagra could be prevented by an appropriate diet without any alteration in hygiene or sanitation.

Simultaneously with his epidemiological studies, Goldberger carried out a series of trials in which he inoculated himself and volunteers from his research team with the secretions and excretions of pellagrinous patients (152). In no instance could the transmission of pellagra be demonstrated, so that these experiments failed to confirm the infective hypothesis.

By this time, influenced by developments in the study of beriberi, Goldberger had begun to see the problem in terms of the deficiency of a specific nutritional factor. He set out to test this theory by a study in which a group of volunteers at a prison farm, where pellagra was unknown, were kept on a diet deficient in animal protein food. The remaining convicts on the farm served as control subjects, all non-dietary factors being held constant. In half the experimental subjects, well-marked skin eruptions, typical of pellagra, had appeared by the end of the fifth month.

Before proceeding to community studies, Goldberger scrutinized the methods used by the Thompson-McFadden Commission, which had only recently arrived at conclusions so different from his own. A number of possible sources of error could be discerned. Dietary data had been based on interviews with patients, which Goldberger considered unreliable. There had been failure to take into account the seasonal fluctuation of pellagra. Finally, case-definition had been ambiguous, so that it was not clear whether the survey had included quiescent as well as active cases.

In a survey designed to avoid these errors, Goldberger and his co-workers examined the diet, economic conditions and sanitation of seven cotton-mill villages in South Carolina, an area of endemic pellagra, and related each of these factors to the incidence of the disease (156). Cases were clearly defined for operational purposes: only those with symmetrical bilateral eruptions of recent onset, and therefore active, were to be included. Incidence was assessed by means of bi-weekly house-to-house search in the villages concerned, during the period from mid-April to the end of the year. Dietary intake was to be assessed not by direct questioning of the local inhabitants, but from the sales records of the stores where they purchased their food. For this purpose, a fifteen-day sample period was chosen immediately preceding or coincidental with the sharp seasonal increase of pellagra in late spring, a point regarded as crucial to the success of the study. The food intake of those households affected with pellagra was then compared with the corresponding intake for the remaining households. Various dietary elements were examined in turn, all other factors being held constant, in a series of tables which demonstrated that deficiencies of either meat or milk could affect the incidence of pellagra. The method is exemplified by Tables III and IV.

The investigators concluded that there was no quantitative difference between pellagrin and non-pellagrin diets and that the merely quantitative statements about diet with which most previous workers had been content had been wholly misleading. They showed that restriction of animal protein foods predisposed to pellagra and that there was a marked inverse correlation between supplies of milk and fresh meat and the incidence of the disease. Hence, important practical measures of prevention and control were suggested, namely to increase the availability of milk, es-

TABLE III

PELLAGRA INCIDENCE BY HOUSEHOLD MILK SUPPLY: SEVEN VILLAGES
OF SOUTH CAROLINA, 1916*

Household Supply of Milk in Quarts Per Adult Male Unit† for a 15 Day Period	Total Number of Households	Number of Households Affected With Pellagra	Percent of Households Affected With Pellagra
All amounts	464	46	10.0
Less than 1.0	103	23	22.3
1.0 – 3.9	63	5	7.9
4.0 – 6.9	90	7	7.8
7.0 – 12.9	102	7	6.9
13.0 – 18.9	67	4	6.0
19.0 and over	39	0	0.0

*This table is restricted to the households of cotton mill workers whose supply of fresh meats was less than one pound per adult male unit per fifteen day period, classified according to the household supply of milk, per adult male unit for a fifteen day period between April 16 and June 15, 1916.
†Adult male unit requirement calculated on the Atwater scale of food requirements.

TABLE IV

PELLAGRA INCIDENCE BY HOUSEHOLD FRESH MEAT SUPPLY: SEVEN
VILLAGES OF SOUTH CAROLINA, 1916*

Household Supply of Fresh Meats in Pounds Per Adult Male Unit† for a 15 Day Period	Total Number of Households	Number of Households Affected With Pellagra	Percent of Households Affected with Pellagra
All amounts	435	45	10.3
Less than 1.0	282	40	14.2
1.0 – 2.9	114	4	3.5
3.0 and over	39	1	2.6

*This table is restricted to the households of cotton mill workers whose supply of fresh milk was less than seven quarts per adult male unit per fifteen day period, classified according to the household supply of fresh meats per adult male unit, for a fifteen day period between April 16th and June 15th 1916.
†Adult male requirement calculated on the Atwater scale of food requirements.
Source: Adapted from Terris (450).

pecially by increasing cow ownership and of fresh meat by introducing all-year-round meat markets.

Thus, by their outstanding work, Goldberger and his colleagues provided the key to the problem of pellagra prevention and control, even though the exact nature of the dietary deficiency remained unknown during his lifetime. All his investigations were carried out with exemplary thoroughness and pertinacity, while the combination of clinical, epidemiological and experimental techniques which he employed stands as a model for collaborative research.

During the present century, epidemiologists have been confronted more and more by problems for whose solution the simple model of a single causative agent is unhelpful. Even in the field of infectious epidemiology, they are now concerned with virus diseases in whose spread individual susceptibility is a crucial factor (55). The renewal of interest in epidemiology has arisen chiefly, however, from the realization that its methods can be applied to the study of non-communicable conditions such as coronary artery disease, peptic ulcer and bronchial carcinoma, as well as to other causes of death and disability such as traffic accidents. Throughout this field of research—and not least in respect of mental disorders—questions of susceptibility, though complex, must be accorded the highest importance. Hence, the epidemiologist's attention has become concentrated less upon the "agents" of disease, more upon the interaction between "host" and environment.

One of the first major studies of this kind was undertaken, not by a medical investigator, but by the French sociologist Emile Durkheim, whose treatise on suicide (102) represents a milestone of psychiatry, as well as of his own newly founded discipline.

DURKHEIM ON SUICIDE: THE SOCIOLOGICAL APPROACH

At the end of the 19th Century, when Durkheim undertook his enquiry, national suicide statistics were scanty and simple correlation techniques unknown. Although his research was based primarily on the published statistics of European countries, he also carried out a personal analysis of the case-records of some 26,000 suicides in France. His definition of suicide was succinct: "all cases of death resulting directly or indirectly from a positive or negative act of the victim himself, which he knew would produce the result." Having estimated suicide mortality rates based on the ratio of known suicides to population size, he found them remarkably constant for any one nation over relatively long periods of time: a point illustrated in Table V.

TABLE V

RATE OF SUICIDES PER MILLION INHABITANTS AND RANK ORDER FOR SUICIDE OF THE DIFFERENT EUROPEAN COUNTRIES

	Quinquennial Period		
Country	1866-70	1871-75	1874-78
Saxony	293 (1)	267 (1)	334 (1)
Denmark	277 (2)	258 (2)	255 (2)
Prussia	142 (3)	134 (4)	152 (4)
France	135 (4)	150 (3)	160 (3)
Bavaria	90 (5)	91 (6)	100 (6)
Sweden	85 (6)	81 (7)	91 (7)
Austria	78 (7)	94 (5)	130 (5)
Norway	76 (8)	73 (8)	71 (9)
England	67 (9)	66 (10)	69 (10)
Belgium	66 (10)	69 (9)	78 (8)
Italy	30 (11)	35 (11)	38 (11)

Source: Durkheim (102).

Durkheim concluded that for any given society the suicide rate was a distinctive, relatively unchanging characteristic: a function of the total culture. In his view, suicide was essentially a collective phenomenon and personal factors were of secondary importance. Each society, he believed, had what amounted to a collective disposition towards suicide, which remained constant so long as the basic cultural patterns were unchanged and which formed part of the individual's social environment, exercising a powerful influence upon him. Any degree of estrangement of the individual from the society in which he lived tended to produce a state of anomie which predisposed him to suicide.

Suicide rates in Catholic countries such as Spain and Portugal were noted to be consistently lower than in those such as Germany where Protestants predominated. Recognising, however, that it would be rash to accept such figures uncritically because of the many uncontrolled variables, Durkheim went on to compare the suicide rates for different religious groups within the various countries. Thus, he examined the rates for eight Bavarian and thirteen Prussian provinces, and also for the Swiss Cantons, which had widely differing proportions of Catholic and Protestants. In all three countries he confirmed that "everywhere without exception, Protestants showed far more suicides than followers of other confessions." His results for the Bavarian Provinces are shown in Table VI.

TABLE VI
SUICIDE RATES FOR THE BAVARIAN PROVINCES, 1867-75*

Provinces With Catholic Minority (Less Than 50%)	Suicides Per Million Inhabitants	Provinces With Catholic Majority (50% to 90%)	Suicides Per Million Inhabitants	Provinces More Than 90% Catholic	Suicides Per Million Inhabitants
Rhenish Palatinate	167	Lower Franconia	157	Upper Palatinate	64
Central Franconia	207	Swabia	118	Upper Bavaria	114
Upper Franconia	204			Lower Bavaria	19
Average	192	Average	135	Average	75

*The population below 15 years has been omitted
Source: Durkheim (102).

By this technique of replicated studies, Durkheim was able to study the association between suicide and religious persuasion, while holding all other variables constant: essentially the same method which had been used by Snow and Goldberger in their studies of disease. Durkheim had to rely much more heavily than these workers on previously available statistics; nevertheless, his labours were prodigious and his results stand as a testimony to what can be achieved in this field with even the simplest statistical tools.

With the benefit of hindsight, it is easy to see Durkheim's work as a landmark in the development of social psychiatry: as the precursor, indeed, of all those studies of the ecology of mental disorder which came to occupy so prominent a place in psychiatric research half a century later. At the time, however, it appeared isolated from the main body of research in this field, which still centred on the analysis of institutional statistics.

THE STATISTICS OF INSANITY

The earliest statistical studies of mental illness attempted to estimate its prevalence in national populations from the returns of lunatic asylums. An outstanding pioneer was Esquirol who, besides presenting the findings of his own survey of French asylums, reviewed the available data from a number of countries and estimated the prevalence of mental illness as a rate for each population (110). Keenly aware of the problems of bias attendant upon sampling procedures, Esquirol warned against uncritical acceptance of any statistics on the subject, including his own.

The nineteenth century saw a number of important contributions to the statistics of insanity, including those of William Farr (117) and John Thurnam (452) in England, and of Isaac Ray (387) in the United States. The United States Bureau of the Census began to enumerate the mentally sick in 1850, and within thirty years were publishing detailed and reliable data (303). While some contemporaries were highly sceptical of the value of these early mental hospital statistics (24), they have since been put to good use in retrospective studies such as those by Goldhammer and Marshall in Massachusetts (157) and by Astrup and Ødegaard in Norway (11).

From the earliest reports, one finds in the commentaries a note of dissatisfaction with the limitations of institutional returns. Already, in the seventeenth century, the London haberdasher and vital statistician, John Graunt, was complaining that the numbers of the insane were underreported: "I fear many more than are set down in our Bills of Mortality, few being entered for such, but those who die at Bedlam. . . ." (165). Linked with this theme, and like it stemming from the desire to put the statistics to practical use, was a recurring preoccupation with *trends* in the incidence of mental disorder. Esquirol in France (110) and Maudsley in England (310) examined the apparent increase, both concluding that it was due to an improvement in treatment facilities rather than to a true rise of prevalence. Daniel

Hack Tuke (459), who conducted a careful analysis of hospital statistics in the 1870s, distinguished clearly between the prevalence and the inception of mental disease:

> The first error into which everyone falls who is not accustomed to the sources of fallacy which beset such figures is taking the actual number of lunatics reported to be under care at any given time as representing the liability of a people to insanity, whereas the only certain proof of this liability is to be found in the numbers who become insane. In other words, the existing lunacy at any period is no indication of the occurring lunacy.

Tuke emphasized that the "enormous accumulation" of mental hospital residents which had occurred in the mid-nineteenth century was not necessarily indicative of a rising incidence of mental illness, but was related rather to social changes, including the building of large asylums. Nevertheless, regarding the numbers of *admissions* to mental hospital as an index of inception, Tuke found it "impossible to deny that there is reason to fear some real increase."

Throughout these years, community surveys were few and far between. Among the earliest were those carried out in Norway, where in 1825 a royal commission was issued to enquire into the conditions of the insane, and to consider measures for their amelioration. Ten years later, a second survey was undertaken, this time in conjunction with a population census. In 1845, a third enumeration was made, together with a survey of the blind, the deaf and dumb, and the lepers. In the towns, this work was undertaken by the magistrates and chief officers; in the rural areas by the parish priests, curates and schoolmasters. Not surprisingly, some diagnostic confusion ensued; nevertheless, in all these surveys it proved possible to enumerate the main diagnostic categories then recognized. Table VII summarizes the 1835 findings, probably the most reliable.

Shortly after the last of these surveys, a community enquiry exceptional both in the sophistication of its methods and the intensity of its case-finding procedure was made in Massachusetts (440). In addition to the use of key informants such as the clergy, overseers of the poor, superintendents of hospitals and masters of

TABLE VII
PREVALENCE OF INSANITY IN NORWAY, 1835

Type of Disorder	Urban		Rural	
	Male	Female	Male	Female
Mania	57	61	306	299
Melancholia	35	45	269	286
Dementia	35	26	226	233
Idiotia	49	34	836	779
All mental disorders	176	166	1,637	1,597
Total population	61,459	67,543	523,922	541,903
Insanity rate per 1,000 population	2.86	2.46	3.12	2.95

Source: Holst (206).

prisons and almshouses, a detailed questionnaire was submitted to every physician practising in the state. As a result, the number of known lunatics and idiots rose from 1,512 to 3,719, an increase of 150 percent. Thus, in its findings as in its methods, the Massachusetts survey foreshadowed the more comprehensive investigations of our own day.

It was not long before reported variation in the statistics of insanity began to be related to local environmental conditions. Bucknill and Tuke (52), observing that insanity rates were higher in urban than in rural areas, speculated on the possible reasons. White (467) claimed that the incidence of insanity varied directly with population density, a fact which he attributed to the greater strain of competitive living in the towns. MacDermott (291) noted wide variation in the prevalence of insanity in Great Britain, both topographically and in some instances locally over the course of two or three generations; such changes he thought unlikely to be explained in terms of hereditary transmission. Nonetheless, it was a preoccupation with genetic factors which was to dominate this field of research increasingly in the early twentieth century.

EARLY RESEARCH IN POPULATION GENETICS

At the time that Kraepelin was working on his classification of the major psychoses, some of his colleagues and pupils were already engaging in community studies. Naecke (342) examined the family history of asylum inmates and Jost (220) those of a sample of healthy people. The work of these and other members of the Munich school has since been reviewed by Strömgren (447), who has emphasized both its historical interest and its value in demonstrating the many pitfalls of method. Later German investigators developed more refined techniques: Rüdin (407) was among the first to employ an unselected patient sample in his studies of morbid risk among the families of schizophrenic patients. Luxenburger (228) used a random sampling procedure to select control subjects from the general population, while Klemperer (244) developed the cohort study in order to compute expectancy rates for mental illness in an urban population. All these workers made valuable contributions to the development of research method, even though in their own studies they were handicapped by major difficulties of classification, sampling and case-detection.

Problems of classification and diagnosis are most easily solved when the mental disorder under enquiry has well-marked physical concomitants, or some associated biological "marker." A strongly familial distribution obviates most of the difficulties of sampling and case-detection, especially in the case of uncommon diseases and those for which a pattern of hereditary transmission can be discerned. The paradigm of such conditions is Huntington's Chorea, which has been a rewarding subject for population genetic studies since its classic description one hundred years ago (210).

One of the largest and most comprehensive surveys of Huntington's Chorea was undertaken in New England by Elizabeth Muncey of the Eugenics Record Office (86). Data were collected by personal observation and questioning of choreics, both in and out of institutions, from hospital and local authority records, from the memory of relatives and neighbours and from the genealogical and town histories with which New England was well-provided. A total of 962 cases was identified on four major pedigree charts, and the medical histories of over 3,000 non-choreic relatives were also examined. The results were valuable in shedding light on several aspects of the natural history of the disease: the existence of different subgroups or "biotypes"; the high prevalence of affective psychosis; the association with alcoholism, suicidal tendencies and possibly with other neurological disorders, including epilepsy; the extensive social consequences. It proved possible to chart the spread by migration of the disease from Long Island Sound westward as far as California, and to relate the origin of all the cases to four nuclear families:

> All these evils in our study trace back to some half-dozen individuals, including three brothers, who migrated to this country during the 17th Century. Had these half-dozen individuals been kept out of this country much of the misery might have been saved.

The task of tracing genetic transmission is essentially similar to that of the clinical epidemiologist investigating an epidemic disease: only the time-scale is different. Even today, a disease such as Huntington's Chorea is more appropriately studied in regions where it is endemic, by the methods of clinical epidemiology, than by systematic prevalence surveys of the general population. Most psychiatric disorders, however, are much more widely distributed, so that the techniques of statistical epidemiology are required: methods of sampling and systematic case-identification then become crucial. The application of sampling methods to the study of mental disorders followed naturally on their development in social survey research (332). Case-identification remains a thorny problem, as we shall see: it was not by chance that the first reliable prevalence figures in psychiatry were obtained in the field of mental retardation, where alone standardized, reliable test procedures were available. For this reason, the work of E. O. Lewis may be taken as the next important landmark in the development of epidemiological psychiatry.

LEWIS' SURVEY OF MENTAL SUBNORMALITY

Lewis set out to estimate the prevalence of mental subnormality in England and Wales as part of an official enquiry into the needs for special medical and educational services (278). He selected for examination six areas, each with a population of about 100,000, which he believed to be representative of the country as a whole. They comprised a metropolitan suburb, a cotton town in

Northern England, a mining and steel engineering area, a prosperous farming area, an agricultural market town and surrounding area of poor farm land in the South West, and, finally, a Welsh rural area with a relative preponderance of the aged and female. Lewis took care to ensure that these areas were not named, a standpoint which has been criticized on the basis that it is difficult for subsequent investigators to confirm or modify the results of his study (172). There can be little doubt, however, that his approach went a long way towards eliminating the errors of bias committed by earlier workers.

This study also provides one of the best examples of the use of key informants. In gathering information, Lewis made use of school teachers, local mental deficiency officers, child welfare clinic personnel, health visitors and district nurses. His methods of case-finding differed according to the age-group under investigation. All school children below nine years of age reported by their teachers to be educationally or developmentally retarded were personally examined by Lewis. On the other hand, older children with low school achievement were first given a group intelligence test and those with low scores then interviewed individually, as were all epileptic and paralysed children.

Detection of subnormality both in adults and among preschool children was less systematic and its thoroughness depended largely on the organisation of social surveys in the areas concerned, with key informants playing an important role.

Case-definition was clearly stated by Lewis in terms of the then official British classification into idiots, imbeciles and the feeble-minded. These categories were based on relatively objective measures of the degree to which the individual could protect and look after himself, manage his affairs or benefit from normal school instruction. The diagnosis of feeble-mindedness is today considered to be largely a function of the prevailing socio-cultural environment, but Lewis' figures for the severer grades of subnormality have stood the test of time remarkably well, and indeed have been used as a basis for estimating changes in prevalence (159).

This investigation also provides an intriguing example of the way in which a prevalence survey undertaken for administrative purposes can incidentally throw light on aetiological factors. In analysing his data, Lewis found evidence of an association between the severity of defect and the type of home background of the child, a finding summarized in Table VIII.

TABLE VIII

DEGREE OF MENTAL RETARDATION IN CHILDREN, BY TYPE OF HOME BACKGROUND

Type of Home Background	Feeble- minded	Grade of Retardation Imbecile	Idiot	All Grades
	%	%	%	%
Superior	1.2	5.9	9.5	2.4
Good	10.1	23.7	23.0	13.2
Average	27.0	36.2	40.5	29.3
Poor	36.5	19.5	21.6	32.7
Very poor	25.2	14.7	5.4	22.3
Total	100.0	100.0	100.0	99.9
No. of children	2,091	419	94	2,604

Source: Adapted from Lewis (278).

This observation led Lewis to postulate the existence of a relatively mild, "subcultural" type of defect, as distinct from the more severe, biologically determined types. His suggestion was taken up by later workers, notably Penrose in his Colchester survey (371); as a result, a dichotomy was established: on the one hand, severe subnormality with a high frequency of neurological signs and a normal socio-economic distribution; on the other, relatively mild subnormality with little or no excess of physical handicaps but preponderance of poor, disorganized home backgrounds. The dichotomy is an oversimplification, inasmuch as we now recognize that biological and socio-cultural hazards to mental development are interrelated. Nevertheless, Lewis' findings represented an important forward step in research on mental subnormality.

During the 1930s, there was a notable increase in the frequency of statistical surveys of mental disorder. The more detailed and comprehensive were of value in drawing attention to the importance of demographic factors such as age, sex, race, marital state, area of residence and geographic mobility (90, 263, 303). At the same time, a growing sociological influence was apparent in those studies which linked urban living conditions to the incidence of suicide (62) and of psychosis (116). Most of the findings, being based on hospital records, related more directly to the utilization of psychiatric services then to true prevalence.

Information on prevalence in the general population remained fragmentary throughout this period. Area surveys were few and, because of the lack of standardized tests or diagnostic procedures, their findings tended to be of low reliability. As a rule, estimates for the major psychoses were more accurate than those for minor forms of mental disorder. Thus, surveys in Germany, Denmark and the United States yielded fairly comparable rates for the psychoses, but not for the neuroses (46, 446, 68).

Following the Second World War, this field of research expanded rapidly. In 1949, the common ground of epidemiology and psychiatry was defined at a conference of workers from both specialties (327). At this point, the historical background of epidemiological psychiatry merges into the foreground of its modern development. In the light of work published in the past twenty years, it is now possible to identify the outstanding problems of method, to define the scope of epidemiology in the study of mental disorders, and to begin to discern the probable directions of future research. It is to these considerations that the succeeding chapters are devoted.

Chapter Two

PROBLEMS OF RESEARCH METHOD

THE PROBLEMS of method encountered in epidemiology vary to some extent with the nature of the disease under scrutiny and its mode of occurrence in populations. Localized outbreaks of communicable disease call for the methods of clinical epidemiology to uncover their origins and modes of spread. This approach is not altogether irrelevant in psychiatry, a point which has already been made with regard to early genetic studies, and will be taken up more fully in Chapter 4. In general, however, mental disorders must be placed in the ranks of endemic disease, whose investigation demands the techniques of statistical epidemiology. It is to a consideration of these techniques that the present chapter is devoted.

The basic aims of any investigation in this field are to establish the prevalence and inception rates of disease, and to test for variations in the rates among defined subgroups of the population at risk. To achieve these aims, the investigator must undertake a series of steps. First, he must select a research strategy which is appropriate to the enquiry, and feasible in economic and logistic terms. Secondly, he must define the survey population and, if it be large, choose a means of securing a representative sample. Thirdly, he must formulate an operational definition of the disease under enquiry which is so precise and unambiguous as to ensure accurate case-identification. Fourth, he must locate and identify all cases of the disease by means of a valid diagnostic technique. Finally, he must express his findings in a manner which will permit replication, and comparison with other surveys. Each of these steps may give rise to difficulties both of concept and of method.

THE RESEARCH STRATEGY

The epidemiologist has available to him a range of techniques from which to select that most appropriate to his needs. The exercise of this choice may be expressed most simply in the form of a series of alternatives, thus:

1. observational	vs	experimental techniques;
2. retrospective	vs	anterospective surveys;
3. cross-sectional	vs	longitudinal surveys;
4. probability sample, or whole population surveys	vs	controlled studies.

In practice, the range of possibilities is not nearly as wide as this framework suggests. Four of the theoretical permutations can be ruled out, since by definition experimental studies cannot be retrospective; others are of little practical significance. The choice is likely to be governed by the purpose of the enquiry, the nature of the disease (and hence its course, duration and distribution), and the resources of the research team. Surveys sponsored by public health authorities will be concerned as a rule with the prevalence of disease at one or more points in time; those which attempt to estimate individual risk and establish prognosis must do so by means of cohort or follow-up studies; those concerned with aetiology will focus on the rate of inception, or appearance of new cases in the population. Confusion is liable to occur only if the investigator fails to distinguish clearly between the different strategies and sets up a research design which does not correspond to any one of them.

DEFINITION OF THE POPULATION

In planning his survey, the investigator must clearly define the population he proposes to study, so that case-finding techniques may be uniformly applied and accurate morbidity rates may be calculated. One term of any such definition must stipulate the geographical boundaries of the population. Where these are regional or local, rather than national, they should as far as possible coincide with administrative boundaries, so that the available official statistics can be utilized. In this context, electoral districts or census tracts are commonly employed because they provide a nominal roll of adult residents, systematically recorded by dwelling and street.

The choice of survey population is a question for the research strategy: as such it will depend on the type of disorder being investigated and the sources of information to be tapped. The choice will be made partly on economic grounds: surveys based on routine administrative data can be of national or state dimensions; those which rely on information gathered at first-hand, being inevitably more onerous and expensive, must as a rule be limited to relatively small areas. The problems of national coverage which so greatly exercise market research and social survey statisticians are seldom of great concern to medical survey workers, morbidity surveys not being feasible on the same scale.

An exception is provided by the type of health survey in which a sample of the national population is selected for interview by trained research assistants using a structured schedule or check-list of medical complaints. Periodic sampling of this kind has been undertaken by health survey teams in a number of countries. An outstanding example in the psychiatric field is the mental health opinion survey carried out some years ago in the United States (176). To learn something about popular attitudes to mental health and psychiatric agencies, the Joint Commission on Mental Illness and Health asked the University of Michigan Survey Research Center to make a nationwide interview survey. A probability sample of 2,500 Americans living at private addresses was so selected as to represent the nation in terms of age, sex, educational achievement, income, occupation and area of residence. Since only 8 percent of the sample refused interview, the respondents were deemed to be "an accurately proportioned miniature of the normal, stable adult population of the United States."

While there can be little doubt that the response was more representative of the nation as a whole than one can normally expect from a health survey, the findings illustrate the weakness of this approach unsupported by clinical examination or judgment. The structured interview included a list of twenty questions about medical complaints, several of which could be considered relevant to mental health, for example:

1. Do you ever have any trouble getting to sleep, or staying asleep?

2. Have you ever been bothered by nervousness, feeling fidgety or tense?
3. Are you ever troubled by headaches or pains in the head?
12. Are you ever bothered by nightmares?
14. Do your hands ever tremble enough to bother you?
15. Are you troubled by your hands sweating so that you feel damp and clammy?
19. Have you ever felt that you were going to have a nervous breakdown?

When the responses to all twenty items were subjected to factor analysis, four main factors appeared to account for the response patterns of both sexes: these were labelled Psychological Anxiety, Physical Anxiety, Physical Health and "Immobilization." While this technique permitted the findings to be set out in terms of the distribution of scores for the four factors, it could provide no meaningful data on the prevalence of neurotic illness, or even of symptoms, among the survey respondents; hence its value for medical planning seems dubious.

Such limitations are now widely recognized as a major defect of health surveys carried out by lay interviewers. In their retrospective account of the British Survey of Sickness, Logan and Brooke (286) commented frankly on this aspect:

> Foremost among the factors for which the Survey of Sickness has been adversely criticised has been that the information it produced was obtained from patients themselves and not from medical sources. As every doctor knows, the accounts which many patients give of their present and past illnesses are often unreliable, and not to be taken at face-value; and whilst such information can be immediately interpreted and used by the doctor as he interrogates and examines his patient, no such medical editing of the patients' diagnostic statements has a place in the methodology of the Survey of Sickness. Though patients no doubt described their complaints correctly and did their best to report diagnoses that their doctor had mentioned, it is probable that non-medical enquiries about illnesses produce less accurate diagnostic information than that obtained from medical practitioners or from any form of medical record prepared by them.

In view of these shortcomings, the writers concluded that health surveys should be regarded as a supplement, rather than as an alternative, to the systematic collection of medical data. In future surveys, they suggested:

> . . . the effect of memory error would be reduced by shortening the period enquired about; questions yielding vague, misleading or otherwise unsatisfactory responses would be eliminated; and attention would be directed to factual questions on which the subject's answer would probably be reliable. . . . The survey method has established itself as a valuable technique in various fields, and it has its place as a method of morbidity ascertainment. It can best make its contribution, however, not as a permanent operation designed to measure the total load of ill-health, its nature, distribution and trends, but to contribute from time to time, as the need arises, particular items of information on illness and its effects that cannot be readily obtained in a routine way.

In the light of such comments, one can readily understand why epidemiologists have placed more weight on the kind of survey in which all members of a population, or a random sample thereof, can be subjected to clinical assessment. The subject of enquiry may, of course, dictate limits other than the geographical: studies of senile or childhood disorders, the diseases of women, and industrial or other occupational diseases constitute obvious examples.

The choice of area will be influenced by local administrative requirements and facilities. Other factors may be relevant; for example, the use of islands with "captive" populations has been a recurring theme in this field of research. The existence of a ready-made sampling-frame may also provide an inducement, as in the psycho-social studies of Welsh mining communities which followed earlier surveys of pneumoconiosis and other forms of physical morbidity (386).

Since any large survey will take weeks or even months to complete, the question of changes in the population at risk must be borne in mind. This factor may be important in psychiatric surveys, there being some evidence that geographically mobile individuals carry an increased risk of mental disorder (305). In ecological surveys, comparisons between the psychiatric rates for different areas must take account of their differences in population turnover.

Some investigators have been able to establish personal contact with every member of a risk-population (37, 111, 177). More often, especially in modern industrial society, the numbers involved are too great and some form of sampling procedure becomes necessary. The essence of modern sampling technique is that the investigator selects a probability sample devoid of bias, so that each member of the population has an equal chance of being included, independent of his relation to any other member. Strictly random techniques may be employed, as with the aid of a book of random numbers (233). A quasi-random technique is often utilized, as for instance the selection of every nth person on a nominal roll. Such methods are acceptable so long as they do not influence the chances of individual selection. That faulty techniques may result in serious bias is well recognized in the field of opinion polls. A case in point is the Literary Digest's notoriously wrong forecast for the 1936 Presidential Election, which was based on a sample restricted to persons listed in telephone directories— an unrepresentative group of the population—and a low response rate. The same considerations apply to morbidity surveys, where at times the fallacies have been equally great.

Time-sampling methods may be subject to bias arising from seasonal fluctuations or even from day-to-day variation: thus, doctors on average will see more alcoholic patients on Mondays than on other days of the week. The dangers of alphabetical sampling were neatly demonstrated by the finding that in England Celtic surnames, commonly beginning with M or O, were associated with blood-group frequencies significantly different from those of the rest of the population (394). While as a rule the representativeness of any given sample is easily tested in terms of age, sex and social class distribution, such relatively subtle types of bias as the above may easily escape detection.

Where the population at risk is very large, or the geographical area extensive, some form of multi-stage sampling procedure may be indicated. In this event, certain areas with known ecological characteristics may be taken as representative and the population of each sampled. In his classic survey of mental deficiency (278), Lewis selected six widely differing areas of England and Wales, including a metropolitan suburb, a cotton-mill town, a mining and steelworks area and contrasting types of rural community; he then used their mean rates of mental retardation to give an index of national prevalence. This commonsense approach has been criticised for its unwarranted assumptions (172). A more sophisticated variant of the same approach may be used where an ecological register is available, as with the standard work of reference on British towns (333).

In the context of a morbidity survey, the first stage of sampling might more appropriately consist of the selection of hospitals, or local lists of a health insurance scheme, were it not for the difficulty of obtaining a random sample of such agencies. In Great Britain, the same problem arises over the sampling of general practitioners, whose lists of registered patients under the National Health Service represent an extremely valuable sampling frame. Since very few investigators have secured a random sample either of doctors or of hospitals, most have had to rely on those institutions and individuals whose cooperation could be gained. There are a number of instances of surveys in which the first stage of sampling has comprised the recruitment of suitable volunteers, while the second stage has involved a random or quasi-random technique (423, 470).

Where social or demographic groupings of the population are markedly unequal, some form of weighted sampling may be required to ensure the inclusion of adequate numbers in each subgroup. The British National Survey of Child Health (97), for example, was based on a stratified sample comprising all children of professional-class parents, and one in three of all other children, born during one week in 1946.

The paramount difficulty of sampling in most community surveys arises not from the method of selection but from the failure of a section of the population to cooperate. Any seriously incomplete coverage due to non-response or refusal must throw doubt on the validity of the findings, since those persons who fail to take part may differ in important respects from the remainder of the sample. The screening of populations for uterine cancer and precancerous change is a case in point, women who attend for cervical smear tests having a lower risk for these conditions than those who fail to attend. The danger of this kind of bias must be taken seriously in psychiatric research, the patient's attitude to survey enquiries being subject to the influence of any mental disturbance. Such a bias may operate in more than one direction, since, as Kessel and Shepherd have remarked,

> . . . a phobic or paranoid patient may, as part of his illness, avoid the doctor as assiduously as the hysteric or hypochondriac consults (240).

The effects of non-response cannot, therefore, be entirely mitigated by the substitution of alternative subjects. The extent of bias caused by non-response can be gauged to the extent that it is possible to compare known characteristics of non-respondents with those of the main survey sample: a general consideration of this technique will be found in standard texts on survey method (332, 486) , but the application to medical surveys in general, and psychiatric surveys in particular, requires great care. Where the failure rate is high, or the nature of the enquiry makes it intrinsically improbable that a random sample can be obtained, the investigator will be wiser to relinquish any claim to representative findings. In this event, a survey which makes use of large numbers of self-selected volunteers may still yield much valuable information, as in studies of human sexual behaviour (242, 243) .

CASE DEFINITION AND CRITERIA

In dealing with chronic, endemic disease, the investigator must have precise, operational definitions which will enable him when in doubt to distinguish between "cases" and "normals." Since clear-cut transitions from illness to health, or from one type of morbidity to another, form the exception rather than the rule, neither the construction nor the application of such definitions will be simple. Both the recognition of illness and the decision to seek help are heavily weighted by socio-cultural factors, which also help to determine the physician's response (223, 320) . The problem is perhaps greatest in psychiatry, where objective signs of disease may be lacking and few valid diagnostic tests exist.

The extensive literature on the definitions of mental illness and mental health serves to illustrate how widely opinion differs on such fundamental issues as the relevance of social functioning

(273, 482) and the importance of cultural expectations (355). Most workers in this field have reached the conclusion that no universally acceptable, unitary definition of mental illness or of its obverse is possible (215, 483). Hence, operational definitions must be carefully considered in the context of each individual research project.

It is remarkable how often the need for some form of case-definition has been neglected. Of twenty-four group investigations reported in the *British Medical Journal* during one year, adequate case-criteria were supplied in only half; seven papers gave imprecise definitions and five none at all. Fletcher and Oldham (121), who cite this example, also give the requirements for a good definition. First, it must be *appropriate* to the study in hand. There would be little point in defining pneumoconiosis in terms of its morbid anatomy, since a case could not then be confirmed ante-mortem: here, the best definition is one based on the radiological appearances. Equally, in a psychiatric survey, definitions should not be based on the underlying psychopathology. Hysterical reaction, for example, is defined by the *APA Diagnostic and Statistical Manual* (9) as follows:

> This neurosis is characterized by an involuntary psychogenic loss or disorder of function. Symptoms characteristically begin and end suddenly in emotionally charged situations and are symbolic of the underlying conflicts. Often they can be modified by suggestion only. . . .
>
> In the conversion type, the special senses or voluntary nervous system are affected. . . . Often the patient shows an inappropriate lack of concern or *belle indifférence* about these symptoms which may actually provide secondary gains by winning him sympathy or relieving him of unpleasant responsibilities. This type of hysterical neurosis must be distinguished from psychophysiological disorders, which are mediated by the automatic nervous system; from malingering, which is done consciously; and from neurological lesions, which cause anatomically circumscribed symptoms.

Hempel (192) has pointed out that such definitions are unsatisfactory for taxonomic purposes, depending as they do in part, not on observable phenomena, but on a number of theoretical premises.

Secondly, the terms of the definition must be so *precise* that the investigator is clearly aware of the features which must be present (and, conversely, those which must be absent) for positive case-identification. Failure to observe this precept has vitiated much research on schizophrenia (16) and, indeed, on other types of mental disorder. Kessel (236) has shown how widely varying prevalence estimates may result from failure to define one's boundaries. In a general practice population, the one-year prevalence rate for psychiatric diagnoses was 50 per 1,000 at risk. If the definition was extended to cover all conspicuous psychiatric morbidity, regardless of formal diagnosis, the rate increased to 90 per 1,000. When conditions with no established structural pathology, such as migraine and functional dyspepsia, were added, the count rose to 380 per 1,000. Finally, the addition of "psychosomatic disorders" such as essential hypertension, asthma and peptic ulcer yielded a total prevalence of 520 per 1,000. Even this figure excluded cases of undoubted physical disease with a secondary psychogenic component.

Thirdly, because many morbid conditions shade imperceptibly into the normal range of health, some artificial boundary or threshold of *severity* is needed for operational purposes. Such a threshold will be most satisfactory if directly related to the degree of associated functional impairment. Thus, limitation of movement provides a simple index of the severity of joint lesions; the distance a patient can walk without stopping is a gauge of occlusive arterial disease. Measures of psychiatric severity are seldom so simple and reliable: more frequently, composite measures based on a number of features of the disorder must be employed. Inconsistent and non-comprehensive classifications may give rise to confusion: if A constitutes the mildest grade, A + B the next, A + B + C the next, and so on, then combinations such as A + C and B + C must be absent, or so rare as to be unimportant.

Difficulties may arise over patients who display unusual symptom-complexes: for example, the predominance of social dysfunction over clinical symptoms in some patients has led community-oriented psychiatrists to posit a distinct "social breakdown syndrome" (173, 299). It is, nonetheless, unusual for hospital-trained psychiatrists to find themselves completely out of their depth when engaged in community surveys. More often, uncertainty arises over those persons who show such mild variants of well-known syndromes that they may be regarded as within the limits of normality. In deciding the lower threshold of morbidity, the introduction of criteria based on functional impairment seems inescapable.

If concise descriptive definitions are often difficult to formulate, the clinically trained investigator can at least call in aid his hospital and practice experience. Observing the resemblance of some people in his survey sample to the patients he sees in his clinical work, he is able in effect to extrapolate his diagnostic criteria beyond their ordinary limits of application. The principal function of an operational definition, therefore, is not to supplant the ordinary diagnostic criteria, but to improve the standard of consistency among medical investigators, and to settle doubt about borderline cases. Case-definition is thus complementary to the standardizing of classification and diagnostic technique.

CASE-FINDING AND CASE-IDENTIFICATION

In order to enumerate all cases of a given disease in any population, two distinct activities must be undertaken: first, the total number of ascertained, or "declared" cases must be calculated; secondly, all unknown, or "undeclared," cases which exist in the population must be detected and added to the total count. According to the type of morbidity and the availability of medical services for its treatment, these two forms of activity may assume greatly varying relative importance; rarely, however, can either be neglected.

The Enumeration of Declared Cases

Until recent years, the chief source of information on the health of populations was provided by officially collected *mortality* data, or "vital statistics." As the focus of interest in modern public health research has swung to chronic, non-infectious disease, so public health workers have become increasingly concerned with the statistics of *morbidity*. Apart from the question of suicide, vital statistics have contributed relatively little to our knowledge of the epidemiology of mental disorder. One notable exception is provided by the use of autopsy findings in estimating the prevalence of chronic alcoholism.

Jellinek (218), a pioneer in the study of alcohol addiction, suggested that the prevalence of severe alcoholism in a population could be estimated from the formula:

$$A = \frac{P.D}{K}$$

where A = number of alcoholics with physical complications
P = percent of cases of cirrhosis attributable to alcoholism
D = total reported cases of cirrhosis found at autopsy
K is a constant (0.695), derived from $\dfrac{C_1.C_2}{100}$
C_1 being the percentage of alcoholics with cirrhosis and C_2 the percentage mortality among alcoholics with cirrhosis.

Unfortunately, the findings of recent surveys have not confirmed the accuracy of rates derived from this formula: in Great Britain, for example, it would imply an overall rate of about 11 per 1,000 in the general population (228), whereas the most reliable survey findings indicate a rate of the order of six to seven per 1,000 for men and only one or two per 1,000 for women (207, 334).

Most prevalence studies based on routine administrative statistics have been limited to the enumeration of patients in psychiatric hospitals. In surveys of this type, mental illness is defined, explicitly or implicitly, as a psychological disturbance severe enough to require hospital admission and care. Under certain conditions—notably where the number of psychiatric beds is commensurate with the community's needs—this method can be expected to give a fair approximation to the number of severely disturbed individuals in the population. Ødegaard, for example, has contended that all but an insignificant fraction of schizophrenic patients will be admitted to hospital at some stage in the course of their illness, so that rates based on admission and bed-occupancy figures may be taken to reflect the true inception and prevalence of the disease (350). The assumptions underlying this argument have been strongly criticized by a number of workers: Terris, for example, has emphasized the selective bias in mental hospital admission which may affect the diagnostic, ethnic and social composition of institutional populations (451). Certainly, with regard to the neuroses and related minor forms of psychiatric illness there can be no doubt that hospital samples are grossly atypical (75, 239).

In recent years, the trend towards early hospital discharge and maintenance in the community has served to underline the need for statistics from sources outside the mental hospital. A notable development has been the establishment in some areas of cumulative case-registers, which gather information from all local psychiatric agencies, including mental hospitals, community mental health centres and clinics; from public health agencies and, where relevant, from the courts. To be an effective epidemiological tool, a case-register must sytematically monitor all psychiatric service contacts by the population at risk, including those which take place outside the boundaries of its defined area.

Case-registers are cumulative; that is, they permit information to be collated and stored according to an on-going system. Some cases are thus identified which might well escape detection in a cross-sectional survey; moreover, the careers of individual patients can be followed through their contacts with various psychiatric agencies. Since the population of the area in question can be estimated from local census data, declared morbidity can be estimated in terms of point-prevalence, period-prevalence or inception rates. Trends in the use of services can be ascertained, and the effects of introducing new services observed.

Case-registers can also provide operational measures of the incidence of new cases in different subsections of the population: a function with obvious relevance to aetiological research. A report on the register for Salford, England (4) illustrates the use of such an instrument to provide inception rates for treated psychiatric morbidity. The authors considered their findings encouragingly similar to those of other studies which have provided psychiatric inception rates: notably in New Haven, Connecticut (204) and "Lundby," Sweden (177). The resemblances, they remarked, "can be recognized even in mental hospital data, although social selection for admission to hospital evidently exaggerates some of the trends."

There have been striking similarities between the reported findings of widely distant psychiatric case-registers. A comparative study of register data from Baltimore, Camberwell (London) and Aberdeen (479) showed that the declared illness-rates for all three areas were of the order of one percent of the population at risk on a given census day, plus another one percent making con tact with psychiatric services during the subsequent year. The comparative data are summarized in Table IX. Registers in Rochester, New York, North Carolina and Hawaii have yielded similar rates for declared illness prevalence (14).

TABLE IX
ONE-DAY AND ONE-YEAR PREVALENCE IN THREE URBAN AREAS

Rates Per 100,000 Aged 15+	Baltimore (Whites Only)	Camberwell, England	Aberdeen, Scotland
a. One-day prevalance (census day)	1,156	861	854
b. New episode in year following census day	842	1,190	921
One-year prevalence (a + b)	1,998	2,051	1,775

Source: Wing *et al.* (479)

It would be a mistake to assume that the congruence of reported rates denotes their approximation to the true prevalence of psychiatric disorder. More probably, it simply "says something about the proportion of the gross national product which industrial societies are prepared to devote to specialised services for the mentally ill" (477). Closer scrutiny of the Maryland data and the two British registers reveals, for example, that in Baltimore City new episodes accounted for only 42 percent of the total one-year prevalence, as compared to 58 percent and 52 percent respectively for Camberwell and Aberdeen. The disparity was due principally to a relative excess of long-stay hospital in-patients in the American city: a finding which may reflect differences in the hospital discharge and rehabilitation policies of the different health authorities.

As a case-finding instrument, the psychiatric register has serious limitations. Its usefulness must inevitably depend upon the adequacy of the local psychiatric services; where these are scanty or poor in quality, the value of the register will be correspondingly low. Any register monitors only those cases making contact with specialist agencies and so provides an incomplete coverage of morbidity in the community. It will tend to select conditions with conspicuous abnormality or behaviour disorder, notably psychotic states, while many neurotic illnesses and character disorders escape notice. Those registers which provide a detailed and comprehensive record are relatively expensive, and their findings cannot be extrapolated to other areas. Despite these qualifications, the case-register must be regarded as an important advance in morbidity recording, and one which should make an increasing contribution to the epidemiology of mental disorders.

The Detection of Undeclared Cases

The distinction between "declared" and "undeclared" cases, though convenient for the epidemiologist, is by no means precise. To take an obvious example, many cases of notifiable disease which are diagnosed and treated by physicians never appear in the official statistics. In psychiatry, the situation is complicated by poor standards of diagnostic reliability and by confusion over the boundaries of morbidity. All the evidence suggests that, by the standards of clinical psychiatry, general practitioners and hospital physicians alike tend to underreport mental illness because they fail to recognize a proportion of the cases which present to them. Furthermore, they may implicitly recognize mental or emotional disturbance and, indeed, prescribe treatment for it, without making any formal psychiatric diagnosis. In these circumstances, doubts can arise as to the precise point at which a given case should be deemed "declared." Figure 1 provides a simple schematic model of this situation in the ordinary setting of the medical services; this model is easily transposed to an epidemiological framework.

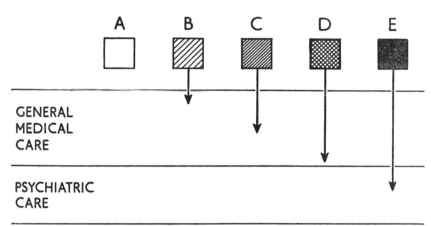

Figure 1. A schematic model of the declaration of psychiatric illness to the medical services. A. No medical contact. B. General medical care only. Psychiatric disorder not recognized. C. General medical care only. Psychotropic drugs perscribed, but no psychiatric diagnosis recorded. D. General medical care only. Psychiatric diagnosis made, but no specialist referral. E. Referral or self-referral to psychiatric agency.

Figure 1 is an oversimplification since it ignores the wide variation between individual doctors' diagnostic and referral rates (423) . Prudence therefore decrees that the research worker should accept as "declared" cases only those patients who have been examined and diagnosed by psychiatrists: viz, Group E in the figure. Groups C and D are better regarded as suspected cases which await confirmation by more detailed examination. Groups A and B clearly cannot be identified in the routine operation of the medical services, but will require special methods.

These considerations underline the general point that the presence of psychiatric disorder is not always easy to ascertain even for medically trained investigators. The problem is by no means peculiar to psychiatry: many of the outstanding diseases of our society require at least a full clinical examination to ensure firm diagnosis, and in addition laboratory or other special tests may be required. The distinguishing feature of psychiatric diagnosis is the weight which, because of the unusual lack of valid tests, must be accorded to the opinion of experienced clinicians. In the words of Blum:

> The interview is the main tool of the psychiatrist—the means he uses to arrive at a diagnosis. It is also the ultimate criterion against which other means for identifying psychiatric disorder are validated. (28).

Few surveys have been based on personal examination of all members of a population, or even of a random sample, by psychiatrists. Occasionally, in small rural communities, it has proved possible to adopt this approach (37, 111, 177), but in the conditions of modern urban society it is hardly feasible. In consequence, a two-stage process of case-identification becomes essential for large-scale field surveys. The first stage is a form of screening procedure which may or may not coincide with the routine work of local medical agencies, and which in effect yields suspected or "potential" cases; the second is a more intensive examination whereby such suspected cases may be verified as confirmed or "actual" cases, or alternatively rejected. Each of these stages will be discussed in turn.

The First Stage: Screening Procedures

Population screening has been defined as:

> ... the presumptive identification of unrecognized disease or defect by the application of tests, examinations or other procedures which can be applied. Screening tests sort out apparently well persons who probably have a disease, from those who do not. A screening test is not intended to be diagnostic. Persons with positive or suspicious findings must be referred to their physicians for diagnosis and the necessary treatment (70).

Screening as a strategy of preventive medicine can thus for practical purposes be equated with the first stage of case-identification. The above definition, however, is more readily applicable to physical than to mental illness, since it assumes the existence of a disease process which can be diagnosed before the onset of symptoms. In psychiatry, the scope for presymptomatic diagnosis is limited by the fact that in the majority of disorders there is no established pathology and no means of objective verification. If, therefore, the concept of screening is to find useful application in psychiatry, it will require modification along the following lines:

> Psychiatric screening is the presumptive identification of previously unrecognised or unreported psychiatric disorder by the application of tests, examinations or other appropriate procedures to defined population samples. Psychiatric screening procedures differentiate between those members of the population who probably have a clinically significant mental or emotional disturbance and those who do not. Such screening tests are not intended to be diagnostic. Persons with positive or suspicious findings will require more intensive examination for definite identification and diagnosis.

To fulfil these conditions, any screening procedure must be relatively cheap, simple to administer, and acceptable to most members of the population at risk. Above all, it must discriminate accurately between those who are sick and those who are well. Any discriminative test can be most simply evaluated in terms of the proportion of individuals correctly classified. The efficiency of a screening test has two components: its *specificity*, or efficiency in detecting valid positives, and its *sensitivity*, or efficiency in detecting valid negatives. An essential prerequisite for the measurement of these variables is the existence of a criterion classification, based on some independent, valid method of discrimination, against which the test results can be judged. In Table X these points are illustrated with reference to a dichotomous classification into "cases" and "normals."

Exactly the same principles apply whether the screening procedure in question is based on a clinical, laboratory or pencil-and-paper test. Indeed, it need not be a test in the narrow sense: routine medical examination, for example, can serve as a screening process, Groups B and C in Figure 1 being an obvious target. Whatever the nature of the screening device, it must be evaluated in terms of its function in a particular enquiry.

Where a choice exists between two or more screening tests,

TABLE X

EFFICIENCY OF A SCREENING PROCEDURE FOR DISCRIMINATING
BETWEEN "CASES" AND "NORMALS"

| | | Criterion Classification | | |
		Cases	Normals	
Test Class-ification	Positive	a	b	a + b
	Negative	c	d	c + d
		a + c	b + d	a + b + c + d

Here, a + b	represents the number of "potential" (suspected) cases revealed by the screening test;
a + c	represents the number of "actual" cases which would be revealed by the validatory procedure;
$\dfrac{a}{a+b}$	represents the *specificity* of the test;
$\dfrac{d}{c+d}$	represents the *sensitivity* of the test;
$\dfrac{a+d}{a+b+c+d}$	represents the overall efficiency of the test.

that one will be preferred which, when measured against the criterion classification, yields the lowest proportion of misclassified individuals: that is, "false negatives" and "false positives" combined. The overall efficiency of a test is not, however, an infallible index of its usefulness as a research tool. This point can be demonstrated by taking the hypothetical example of two tests which, in an experimental situation, misclassify an equal proportion of individuals.

TABLE XI

A COMPARISON OF THE EFFICIENCY OF TWO HYPOTHETICAL
SCREENING PROCEDURES

| | | Criterion Classification | | |
		Cases	Normals	Total
Test A	Positive	92	12	104
	Negative	8	88	96
		100	100	200
Test B	Positive	84	4	88
	Negative	16	96	112
		100	100	200

When validated on 100 cases and 100 normal controls, Tests A and B each produce an overall misclassification of 10 percent. Suppose, however, that each is applied to a population sample of 10,000 which has a "true prevalence" rate of ten per 1,000 at risk for the disorder in question. The criterion classification would divide this population into 100 "actual" cases and 9,900 normals. A simple calculation shows that Test A will select a total of 1,280 persons as potential cases, of whom 92 will subsequently be confirmed. The prevalence rate estimated by this method will be 9.2 per 1,000 at risk, while a total of eight cases will be missed. Test B, on the other hand, will select only 480 potential cases, of which 84 will be confirmed. This method will yield an estimated prevalence rate of 8.4 per 1,000 at risk and will miss a total of 16 cases in the population sample.

Faced with a choice of this kind, the investigator would have to weigh the difficulty of interviewing large numbers of persons at the second stage of the enquiry against the need to procure as accurate as possible a morbidity rate for the population, and to identify as many undeclared cases as possible. In practice, the dilemma of choosing between two equally efficient screening procedures is unlikely to arise. A more common problem is that of deciding on the best threshold, or "cutting score," to adopt when attempting to distinguish between cases and normals by means of a test whose range of scores is unimodally distributed in the population.

A convenient illustration is the use of psychometric tests to discriminate between mentally subnormal and normal individuals. Mental subnormality, or retardation, is essentially a medico-social concept, whose boundaries do not coincide neatly with the distribution of I.Q. scores. The Wechsler Adult Intelligence Scale, for example, has serious limitations as a test for mental retardation (136). Although an I.Q. score of 70 on this scale has been widely accepted as a suitable cut-off point, the available evidence suggests that three-quarters of the persons who score less than 70 are able to lead independent lives and are not regarded in their communities as mentally abnormal. On the other hand, no fewer than 40 percent of clinically subnormal persons have W.A.I.S. scores of 70 or over (59, 348) . Thus, the specificity of the test when used in the general population will be low.

The effect of raising the cutting score to 80 would be to increase the proportion of identified cases from 60 to 80 percent, while at the same time raising the proportion of "false positives" from 1.6 to 8.1 percent of the general population. In this event, the overall efficiency of the test would fall from 0.98 to 0.91. Nevertheless, in a situation where it was important to identify as many as possible of the subnormal members of the population, and where resources were available for clinical examination of large numbers of suspected cases, the higher cutting score might be preferable.

Psychiatric screening methods do not readily lend themselves to any simple, systematic classification. Some make use of formal tests; others rely upon information supplied by key informants. Some are applicable to the general population, others only to special subcategories designated by sex, age-group, occupation or physical health. Some are employed in the setting of medical or para-medical agencies, or of non-medical agencies such as schools or penal institutions, others in the wider community. Clearly, the choice of informant, of agency and of technique will be interdependent and will be governed by the type of mental disorder under review, the sociocultural background of the investigation and the resources of the survey team. Here, only two parameters will be considered: the principal sources of information and the techniques to be utilized.

Sources of Information

In a rural area, where both the density and the mobility of population are low, the survey worker may obtain a great deal of information, within the due limits of confidentiality, from key informants such as general practitioners, public health nurses, school-teachers, clergymen and police. This method, which is most valuable in situations where formal testing would be difficult, has been employed in surveys as far apart as Germany (46) , Tennessee (403) and Formosa (283) .

The key informant is fairly reliable in surveys of the major psychoses, where behavioural disturbances are conspicuous, or of mental retardation, where "lifetime prevalence" is a meaningful concept. He is a poor guide to the prevalence of all the milder, non-psychotic disorders with which Western psychiatry is now concerned. In highly mobile industrial societies, the value of the key informant is in any case much reduced. Of recent years, the emphasis has been placed increasingly on standardized techniques which can be applied to all persons making contact with specified agencies, or to samples of the general population.

Of non-psychiatric medical agencies, the most obviously relevant is the general hospital. Over the past forty years, repeated surveys have confirmed the high prevalence of psychiatric disturbance among patients attending medical out-patient clinics. Table XII summarizes the findings of some of the better-known British and American studies.

Whatever the defects of method in these studies, they have been unanimous in pointing to a high rate of mental disturbance

TABLE XII

PREVALENCE OF PSYCHIATRIC DISORDER AMONG MEDICAL
OUT-PATIENTS

Author	*Place*	*No. of Patients*	*Percent With Psychiatric Disorder*
Buck (51)	(1930) Boston	2,000	36
Reynolds (393)	(1930) Johns Hopkins	935	21
McLean (319)	(1932) Chicago	100	27
Moersch (329)	(1932) Mayo Clinic	500	12
Pearson (367)	(1938) Guy's Hospital, London	1,297	16
Hamman (180)	(1939) Johns Hopkins	500	23
Allan and Kaufman (8)	(1948) Lahey Clinic	1,000	27
Pemberton (370)	(1951) Sheffield, England	146	17
Lewis (276)	(1952) Iowa	151	20
Lewis (277)	(1953) Johns Hopkins	163	49
Davies (88)	(1964) Dulwich, London	100	38
		Total 6,892	Mean 25.7

Source: Davies (88).

among general medical out-patients. Similar findings have been reported from other specialties, notably gynaecology (48), dermatology (415) and venereology (369). These observations have been variously interpreted. Emotionally disturbed persons may as a consequence develop somatic symptoms (302). The presence of physical disease may induce secondary emotional disorder (488). Physical and psychiatric illness may co-exist because of a shared aetiology (49, 98). Persons with a high degree of "neuroticism" may have correspondingly high rates of hospital referral, independent of morbidity (74, 396). Whatever the true cause—and it probably resides in a combination of all these explanations—there can be little doubt that general hospital out-patients constitute an important high-risk group for psychiatric screening.

To a lesser extent, the same principle applies to general practice patients. Indeed, where the bulk of the population is enrolled with general practitioners, as under the British National Health Service, the registered patient-population can provide a very useful sampling frame. In the absence of a state health service, prepaid medical care schemes may be utilized for the same purpose (119), although the coverage provided by such schemes must be seriously incomplete.

Estimates of psychiatric morbidity among general practice patients have varied widely, the most detailed and comprehensive survey of this field yielding a total prevalence rate of 140 per 1,000 adults at risk, or a little over one-fifth of all those who consulted during the survey year (423). Neurotic patients tend to be frequent users of medical services. Hence, the shorter the time-span of observation, the higher the proportion of neurotic illnesses among those who consult: of one consecutive series of over 500 general practice attenders, for example, nearly half had neurotic symptoms (147). Surveillance of a general practitioner's surgery for a fairly limited time-period—say three months—thus provides a relatively efficient method of psychiatric screening. Conversely, those persons who over long intervals of time do not consult their doctors appear to be at low risk for psychiatric morbidity (240).

General practitioners' lists may be used as a framework for *ad hoc* screening surveys. A study of presymptomatic disease in the

40 to 65-year-old age-group, undertaken in a large group practice in southeastern England (104), achieved a 70 percent response, which compares favourably with many public health surveys. The patient's rapport with his family doctor can be of great importance for the success of such projects.

The systematic use of para-medical agencies may also provide a valuable screening system for some types of morbidity. A well-recognized example is the early detection of childhood disorders through routine home-visiting and testing by public health nurses. In a different sphere, social workers and public health nurses have been found at least as effective as doctors in the detection of chronic alcoholism (334, 382). Social agencies concerned with delinquency, child care and welfare of the elderly may all be viewed as potentially valuable for psychiatric screening.

The detection of "potential" cases or high-risk groups may be extended beyond the recognized paramedical services to include other kinds of agencies whose task it is to deal with human predicaments. Thus, Mazer has described the operation of a "para-psychiatric register" on the island of Martha's Vineyard (314). Sources of information include the courts, the school system and the registrar of motor vehicles, as well as the local Department of Welfare. The "parapsychiatric events" which he is thus enabled to monitor are recorded under the following headings:

>   Fine, probation or jail
>   Juvenile delinquency
>   Desertion, separate support or divorce
>   Premarital pregnancy
>   Single car automobile accidents
>   Automobile accidents involving drunkenness
>   Automobile license withdrawal
>   Chronic alcoholism
>   Acute public intoxication with temporary jailing
>   Suicide and homicide
>   School disciplinary problems, high school
>   Psychological counselling, high school
>   School underachievement, high school
>   Welfare recipiency

In addition, all deaths, births, marital dissolutions and mental hospitalizations are recorded in a separate "stressor register."

A system of this kind casts a very wide net: Mazer found that 7 percent of his population had gained at least one entry in the first three months of recording (314). The collection of so much confidential information also raises some delicate ethical problems. Nevertheless, there is every hope that with continuing experience of such a register a carefully selective and efficient technique of case-detection will be evolved.

The use of non-medical agencies need not be confined to this type of monitoring: appropriate agencies may be selected for surveys of various subsections of the general population. The school system is undoubtedly the best framework for surveys of mental retardation (257, 278). Industrial surveys have been used to screen working populations for neurosis (125) and for alcoholism (188). A census of a reception centre for vagrants revealed that one-quarter of the clientele was addicted to alcohol (107). Prison and detention centre populations are other obvious high-risk groups (139, 465).

Selection of Screening Techniques

The case-finding strategy must depend upon the sources of information to be utilized. If the survey population is small and its risk for psychiatric morbidity high, the investigator may dispense with any initial screening procedure and arrange a psychiatric interview with every member of the sample. Such an approach might be appropriate for, say, a survey of sex offenders, or of patients admitted to a poisoning treatment centre (237).

Where the population under review is too large for routine examination, the investigator has a choice of two principal strategies: he can persuade physicians or other professional workers to report to him all suspected cases; alternatively, or in addition, he can introduce some form of standardized test. The latter may consist of a structured or semi-structured ("guided") interview by a research assistant, a rating scale, or a self-administered pencil-and-paper test.

In the past, none of these methods has achieved a high reputation for reliability. Under-reporting by hospital physicians and general practitioners has already been mentioned; the same considerations apply to the use of nurses and social workers as screening agents. Nevertheless, a proportion of the mentally disturbed who would elude detection by any standardized test will be picked out as cases by the doctors or professional helpers to whom they are known. In particular, psychotic individuals who are unwilling to be interviewed or to complete a questionnaire may only be identified by service workers.

There are two broad approaches to screening by means of lay research assistants. In the first, the assistant interviews members of the survey sample with the aid of a structured schedule which is afterwards scrutinized by one or more psychiatrists. The psychiatrist then has the unenviable task of making a clinical assessment without having seen the person concerned. Although diagnosis in the accepted sense may be impossible, some discrimination between "cases" and "normals" can be achieved. The Midtown Manhattan and Stirling County studies (439, 269), which both relied heavily upon this technique, produced findings very different from those of more clinically oriented surveys. Direct comparisons of this kind of indirect assessment with psychiatric interviewing suggest that it has rather low validity (184, 345).

The second approach entails the use of some kind of checklist, rating scale or standardized questionnaire, the responses to which can be scored on simple principles. By means of such an instrument, the research assistant can derive an overall score which, when checked against a predetermined "cutting score," allows each respondent to be classified as a probable case or a probable normal.

The number of psychological scales is large, but the great majority can be dismissed as unsuitable for screening purposes. Personality inventories and attitude scales are inappropriate, since they are not directly concerned with psychiatric disorder. Some techniques which are valuable in the study of individual patients or small groups are too cumbersome and time-consuming for use in large surveys. Psychiatric rating-scales are simple to administer, but most have been designed with severe psychotic illness in mind, and are inapplicable to community studies. Symptom check-lists do not suffer from this disadvantage, but their validity as case-finding instruments seems to be poor (28) ; moreover, their superiority over self-administered questionnaires has not been established.

The self-administered questionnaire—usually in the form of a complaint inventory—is in a number of respects the most effective form of psychiatric screening test. It is cheap, easily administered, quickly completed and scored, and readily acceptable to large sections of the general population. Although theoretical objections can be raised to the use of this method, the acid test must be its success in differentiating between the sick and the healthy. Varying degrees of success have been reported for such instruments as the Cornell Medical Index Health Questionnaire (39, 85), the Health Opinion Survey (269, 296) and Zung's Self-Rating Depression Scale (487). Other instruments constructed primarily for evaluative research are potentially useful in screening; for example, the Johns Hopkins Symptom-Distress Checklist (359) and the Middlesex Hospital Questionnaire (83). So far, however, such methods have had very limited application in epidemiology. Goldberg, following a careful review of the subject, concluded:

> . . . that no scale at present in use has been designed specifically for the task of case-identification, and that most of them do not distinguish between personality traits and symptoms. Very few of them take into account the problems of response bias . . . and in general the more rigorously designed validity studies have produced very disappointing results for the various scales (146).

Current developments in this field will be discussed in Chapter 6.

The Second Stage: Clinical Assessment and Diagnosis

In the Lundby Project, all 2,500 inhabitants of a rural area in Sweden were interviewed by a team of psychiatrists (111) and a decade later the survey was replicated by a single research psychiatrist (177). In most surveys, however, psychiatric examination has had to be restricted to the interviewing of probable cases detected by preliminary screening. Thus, Lewis examined schoolchildren who had done poorly in group intelligence tests (278); Lin in Formosa interviewed persons named by key informants (283), and Mayer-Gross in Scotland adopted the same procedure (313).

Examination by an experienced psychiatrist offers the best hope of valid case-identification. If surveys such as those by Lin and Mayer-Gross, cited above, have yielded unconvincing results (the former, for example, detecting a rate for neurotic illness of only 1.2 per 1,000 at risk), this fact can be attributed largely to defects in the initial screening procedure. Nevertheless, a number of studies have shown that the reliability of diagnosis by clinical psychiatrists can be surprisingly low (113, 251, 417). Awareness of these findings has led to the introduction of more sophisticated techniques, with some consequent improvement in standards. So far, however, the evidence of this improvement remains largely confined to hospital studies. In the words of Foulds,

> ... the earlier and more pessimistic studies of the reliability of psychiatric diagnosis appear to have been superseded by better designed studies which suggest that inter-psychotic: neurotic and intra-psychotic reliabilities are satisfactorily high; whereas intra-neurotic reliabilities are low (123).

Although we have little evidence on the point, it is a fair assumption that inter-neurotic: normal reliabilities, crucial in community surveys, also remain low. Here again, recent developments and prospects for future progress will be reviewed in Chapter 6.

THE MEASUREMENT OF MORBIDITY

Because of the need to compare findings for different populations, epidemiological workers have to make use of standardized measures of mortality and morbidity which can be derived from some generally accepted formulae. Difficulties have arisen in consequence even over mortality data: statistics for morbidity are inevitably less precise and the construction of standardized indices correspondingly more difficult.

In addition to the problems of definition and case-identification outlined above, there are questions concerning the onset, course and duration of illness which may give rise to much confusion. This is especially true of the recurrent, episodic types of morbidity which feature so largely in the psychiatrist's case-material. The findings of surveys covering a year or more will not be directly comparable with those based on a single census day. Base populations which exclude children, or the elderly, will provide rates differing from those for people of all ages. Counts restricted to currently active cases will in general be lower than those which include former, or "inactive" cases. Table XIII illustrates how some of the better-known psychiatric surveys have differed in their coverage and their reported prevalence rates.

More direct evidence of the effect on reported prevalence of the length of observation is provided by a longitudinal study of a population cohort (77). Over a period of seven years, the mean annual psychiatric prevalence was 60 per 1,000 males at risk and 172 per 1,000 females at risk. Corresponding rates for the whole survey period were 238 per 1,000 males and 528 per 1,000 females. In other words, the total number of cases reported over seven years was four times the mean annual figure for men and three times the mean annual figure for women.

This study also demonstrated the problem of defining new cases, and hence of establishing true inception rates. The number of new cases reported during the survey period fell steadily for the first three years among the males at risk and for the first five years among the females at risk. Clearly, if psychiatric disorders ran a discrete, continuous course and all members of the population were equally susceptible, one would expect to find no change in the inception rates for a large population cohort, except for a small rise due to the general effect of ageing. In practice, however, "new" cases, operationally defined, will almost always include some which are really recurrences among susceptible persons.

The indices of morbidity appropriate for any given survey will depend upon the research aims. Public health administrators will be most interested in the *prevalence* and *distribution* of disease in the general population, and in evidence of changing morbidity patterns. Scientific research workers will be more concerned with the rates of *inception*, or appearance of new cases of disease. Oper-

TABLE XIII

COMMUNITY SURVEYS OF PSYCHIATRIC DISORDER: EXTENT AND REPORTED
PREVALENCE RATES

Author	Place	Date of Survey	Period Covered	Age— Range	Rate Per 1,000 at Risk Mental Disorders	Psychoses
Rosanoff (399)	Nassau	1916	one day	all ages	36.4	—
Cohen & Fairbank (68)	Baltimore	1933	one year	over 15	44.5	8.2
Lemkau et al. (271)	Baltimore	1936	one day	over 10	60.5	6.6
Roth & Luton (403)	Tennessee	1935-1938	one day	all ages	46.7	4.9
Bremer (37)	Norway	1940-1945	five years	all ages	193.5	14.3
Lin (283)	Formosa	1946-1948	one day	all ages	10.8	3.8
Eaton & Weil (105)	Hutterite communities	1950	three months	15 & over	16.7	4.7
Trussell & Elinson (457)	New Jersey	1951-1955	one day	all ages	138.0	2.0
Srole et al. (439)	Midtown Manhattan	1952-1958	one day	20-59	233.0	—
Leighton et al. (269)	Stirling County	1951-1962	one day	adult	234.0	—
Shepherd et al. (423)	London	1961-1962	one year	15 & over	139.6	5.8

Sources: Plunkett and Gordon (379); Lin & Standley (284).

ational research on the medical services may focus on numbers of *illness episodes,* or *spells of medical care,* rather than on numbers of persons affected. Similarly, industrial or health insurance studies may set out to measure rates of *disability,* or of *sickness-absence.*

Considerations of this kind led a British official committee on the subject (388) to recommend the use of nine principal indices, as follows:

1. Inception rate (spells) :

$$\frac{\text{Number of spells of sickness starting in a defined period}}{\text{Mean number of persons exposed to risk in that period}}$$

2. Inception rate (persons) :

$$\frac{\text{Number of persons starting at least one spell of sickness in a defined period}}{\text{Mean number of persons exposed to risk in that period}}$$

3. Period prevalence rate (spells) :

$$\frac{\text{Number of spells of sickness current at some time during a defined period}}{\text{Mean number of persons exposed to risk during that period}}$$

4. Period prevalence rate (persons) :

$$\frac{\text{Number of persons who are sick at some time during a defined period}}{\text{Mean number of persons exposed to risk during that period}}$$

5. Point prevalence rate:

$$\frac{\text{Number of persons sick at some point of time}}{\text{Number of persons exposed to risk at that point of time}}$$

6. Mean duration of each completed spell of sickness
7. Mean duration of sickness per case
8. Mean duration of sickness per person at risk
9. Proportion of total survey period spent sick

In this instance, the primary concern was with industrial sickness absence, a "spell of sickness" being defined as "a period during which a person is sick on one day (or shift) or on each of a consecutive series of days (or shifts)." Indices of the kind listed above can, however, be adapted for surveys based on spells of medical care, or illness-episodes operationally defined. Such a system has the great advantage that it renders possible fairly precise comparisons between the findings of different surveys, as in cross-national studies of psychiatric case-registers (479).

Prevalence surveys of mental disorder have been criticised on the grounds that they take no account of differential mortality rates: that is to say, in any cross-sectional survey the population at risk will comprise only the *surviving* members of each generation. This consideration is most obviously important for geneticists, but has its implications for all aetiological studies. In order to overcome the difficulty, psychiatric morbidity rates are sometimes expressed in terms of the "morbid risk" or disease "expectancy" of an individual at birth. The only sure way of ascertaining the expectancy of any disease in a population is to plot the illness-experience of a representative cohort over the entire period at risk. In view of the formidable nature of the task, it is hardly surprising to find a dearth of anterospective studies of this type. A few brave investigators have tried to chart the morbidity experience of a population cohort retrospectively. The most successful of these studies have dealt with static populations such as that of Bornholm Island (128).

More frequently, indirect methods have been employed to compute morbid risk from the findings of prevalence surveys. In Weinberg's method (389) the total number of cases identified in such a survey is divided by an adjusted population figure based on the number of persons who survive the theoretical period of risk for the disease in question. Thus,

$$p = \frac{a}{b - (b_o + \frac{1}{2}b_m)}$$

where p = morbid risk

a = number of persons affected

b = total survey population

b_o = number who have not yet reached the period of risk for the disease

b_m = number within the age-limits of the risk-period.

The above formula has been criticized on a number of points (250). It does not overcome the problem of differential mortality, and adjustments have been made to try to remedy this defect (29). Furthermore, the notion of a "period at risk" is apt to be misleading. In the case of schizophrenia, for example, the usual definition of the risk-period as the range from 15 to 45 years ignores clinical findings of a relatively high frequency of onset in later life (120, 226).

This review of epidemiological methods has emphasized the many questions which remain to be answered and which, it may be safely assumed, will continue to preoccupy investigators for some years to come. Chapter 6 provides a short review of recent advances in methodology, and an outline of current trends in this field. At the same time, the rapid proliferation of applied research during the past thirty to forty years allows us already to make a provisional definition of the scope of epidemiological techniques in psychiatry. The next three chapters are devoted respectively to administrative, clinical and scientific applications.

Chapter Three

USES OF EPIDEMIOLOGY
I. PLANNING MENTAL HEALTH SERVICES

IN ORDER to assess the service needs of a population, medical administrators must have information about the prevalence, distribution and severity of illness among its members. Equally important for planning purposes is a knowledge of the ways in which morbidity patterns and the utilization of medical services are undergoing change. Epidemiological research can thus be of great help to the administrator, both by supplying him with accurate prevalence data and by the detection and monitoring of new trends. Recently, a third function has been recognized: that of evaluating health services in action.

PREVALENCE AND SERVICE NEEDS

Not the least valuable aspect of prevalence surveys has been their exposure of serious deficiencies in the provision of medical and related services for the mentally disordered. A well-known instance was the mental health survey of Williamson County, Tennessee, in 1938 (404). In addition to a survey of the entire county based on the use of key informants, the investigators mounted an intensive study of three randomly selected areas in which all the residents were interviewed. Not surprisingly, this substudy yielded a much higher psychiatric prevalence than the parent survey, the respective rates being 123.7 and 64.5 per 1,000 at risk. Of more immediate relevance was the finding that the number of patients in mental hospitals could be matched with an almost equal number of similar cases in the community receiving little or no medical attention. The data are summarized in Table XIV.

The table indicates that the total number of persons in need of care and supervision was well over double the number in institutions. The greatest disparity was found among the mentally

TABLE XIV
PSYCHIATRIC DISORDER IN RELATION TO INSTITUTIONALIZATION,
BY ETHNIC GROUP: WILLIAMSON COUNTY, TENNESSEE, 1938

| | Psychiatric Prevalence, per 1,000 Popn. | | |
	White	Coloured	Total
Under institutional care	3.0	4.2	3.3
Mental hospital	2.0	2.3	2.1
Other*	1.0	1.9	1.2
Eligible for institutional care	4.4	3.8	4.2
Mental hospital	2.1	1.2	1.9
School for feeble-minded	2.2	2.6	2.3
Total population	19,000	5,800	24,800

*Comprises schools for feeble-minded, reform schools, special institutions and prisons.
Source: Roth and Luton (404).

retarded, where placements covered less than one-tenth of the need. For the mentally ill, institutional figures represented just over half the total of severe cases. Some confirmation for this claim was provided by a comparison of local mental hospital statistics with those for better-endowed states. Table XV shows that by addition of the non-institutionalized cases, the local rates were brought more into line with national figures.

TABLE XV
MENTAL HOSPITAL RATES FOR WILLIAMSON COUNTY COMPARED
WITH THOSE FOR SELECTED STATES, 1938

Area	No. of Cases	Total Population	Rate Per 1,000
United States	499,879	130,112,785	3.84
Massachusetts	26,751	4,304,977	6.21
New York State	77,416	13,323,204	5.81
Tennessee	6,257	2,863,466	2.19
Williamson County:			
in hospital	52	24,804	2.10
in hospital or eligible for hospital	100	24,804	4.03

Source: Roth and Luton (404).

Attitudes to psychiatric treatment have changed over the past thirty years and today the problem would be posed in different terms; nevertheless if we substitute for "institutionalization" the wider concept of medical and social needs, surveys of this kind continue to serve a useful purpose. Recent British examples can be drawn from the fields of mental retardation, child psychiatry and psychogeriatrics.

A survey of school-age children in one region of England (257) found a rate for severe subnormality (I.Q. below 55) of nearly four per 1,000 at risk; of these, little more than half were known to the health authorities. In Table XVI, the findings have been extrapolated to a standard population of 100,000.

TABLE XVI
ESTIMATED AND DECLARED PREVALENCE OF SEVERELY SUBNORMAL
CHILDREN PER 100,000 TOTAL POPULATION

Age-group:	0–4	5–15	Total
Estimated total	30	66	96
No. known to Mental Health Dept.	4	47	51
Home care only	2	7	9
Home care plus training centre	1	22	23
Hospital or hostel	1	16	17
Other	—	2	2
Estimated no. *not* known to Mental Health Department	26	19	45

Source: Kushlick (257).

Although the hospital and community health services with which the survey was concerned were more advanced than those in Williamson County thirty years earlier, the main conclusion is the same: Table XVI indicates a need for medico-social services much greater than the provision. As a result, new services have been planned for the region, based on the model of the small "family-type" residential unit. In this instance, a prevalence survey constituted the first stage in an on-going research programme which is now proceeding to evaluative studies (258).

Some comparable findings were provided by a survey of neuro-psychiatric disorders among school-age children on the Isle of Wight (412). Of a total of over 2,000 children subjected to a two-stage screening procedure, 2.2 percent were found to have relatively severe psychiatric disturbance, while altogether 6.3 percent were eligible for specialist referral for diagnosis, treatment or advice. In fact, only 0.7 percent were receiving any form of treatment, that is, one in nine of all those for whom it was indicated.

The difficulties of planning services of this kind were illustrated by the finding that only one in six of the disturbed childrens' parents recognized, or were willing to admit, the need for treatment; nevertheless, as the investigators commented, public attitudes on such issues tend to change once new services have been established.

At the other end of the age-range, a survey of psychogeriatric disorders in the industrial city of Newcastle-upon-Tyne (225) showed an even greater disparity between the need and the availability of psychiatric services. The survey sample was selected at random from the electoral register and subjects were interviewed at home; at the same time, a census was taken of patients and residents in mental hospitals, geriatric wards and welfare homes. The results are summarized in Table XVII.

TABLE XVII

ESTIMATED TOTAL PREVALENCE RATES FOR THE MAIN PSYCHIATRIC DISORDERS PER 1,000 POPULATION AGED 65 YEARS OR OVER

	Institutional Cases Per 1,000	Domiciliary Cases Per 1,000	Total Prevalence Per 1,000	Approx. Ratio Domiciliary/ Institutional Cases
Senile and arteriosclerotic dementia	6.8	38.8	45.6	6
Other severe brain syndromes	0.8	9.7	10.5	
Manic-depressive disorder	0.7	12.9	13.6	
Schizophrenia, chronic	(0.2)*	9.7	10.8	(12)
Paraphrenia, late onset	0.9	0.0		
Psychoses, all forms	9.4	71.1	80.5	8
Brain syndromes, mild forms	5.3	51.8	57.1	
Neuroses and allied disorders (moderate/severe forms)	1.9	87.4	89.3	23
Character disorders, inc. paranoid states	0.5	35.6	36.1	
All disorders	17.1	245.9	263.0	14

*Long-stay mental hospital schizophrenics not included
Source: Kay *et al.* (225).

Table XVII does not in itself provide an index of needs and resources; obviously a high proportion, even of the elderly with major psychiatric disorders, would not require institutional care even if beds were available. Nevertheless, the findings of a ratio of six to one between domiciliary and institutional cases of organic brain disease, together with the observed deficiencies in community care facilities, prompted this group of workers to conclude that more services were urgently needed.

Opinions differ as to the value of local area surveys in estimating service requirements. Lapouse has attacked the view that a prevalence survey is a necessary or desirable preliminary to the setting up of each new mental health centre:

> From a practical point of view the community mental health centers will have difficulty for many years to come in saturating their "catchment" areas with enough services to meet the needs of those with severe mental illness (265).

There is considerable force in this argument, as also in Lapouse's criticism of the defects of method in some of the better-known prevalence surveys. It was aimed, however, at a particular historical situation: in a broader context, one can readily envisage a number of situations in which prevalence surveys may be rewarding. A balanced view will consider not only the immediate object of securing reliable morbidity data, but also the further steps whereby prevalence figures are translated into realistic estimates of needs and priorities, administrators are persuaded to base their planning on such estimates and, finally, the plans of administrators are put into effect. Where the later stages are feasible, the first—that of the prevalence survey—may be crucial. Admittedly, examples of area or national surveys as an incentive and guide to planning are still rare, but they do exist. The study of mental retardation by Kushlick, already cited, is a case in point; another is a survey of child autism in Great Britain which has been influential for the planning of special educational services (287).

For local purposes, cumulative case-registers provide a better guide to the need for services than do prevalence surveys, since the course of illness in various subgroups, and the current patterns of contact with medical agencies, can be analysed. Thus, Gardner used the Rochester Register to highlight disparities in the provision of services for middle-class and lower-class districts (134), while in England, data from the Camberwell Register have been used to support the argument for rationalizing local services (477). Case-registers may also be useful for monitoring trends in declared illness.

Certain population subgroups present special problems in the planning of mental health services. Skid row alcoholics, vagrants and the inmates of some state and charitable institutions are at high risk for mental disorder. A census of a London reception centre (107) found that 25 percent of the residents were chemically dependent on alcohol; at least 7 percent had made suicidal attempts; the same proportion had been in prison during the preceding six months, and altogether nearly two-thirds had prison records. Few members of this type of drifting population come into contact with psychiatric agencies, except as the result of imprisonment or social crises. On the basis of such findings, the need for special screening programmes is becoming more widely accepted.

Many members of these high-risk groups are reluctant to seek medical or social help, an attitude which may be a direct expression of mental illness or personality disorder. New ways must be found of bringing therapeutic or preventive measures to bear in this situation. In one experiment on the management of skid row alcoholics (72), the daily routine of a hostel was geared to the requirements of men who for many years had been leading destitute, disorganized lives, punctuated only by intermittent spells in hospital and prison. When methods of persuading such men to accept medico-social care were explored, it became clear that their attitudes to the rehabilitation service were crucial; in the event, a favourable shift of attitude could be achieved most successfully by means of group therapy.

Other subgroups with special needs include the prison population, narcotic addicts, and some kinds of juvenile delinquent. Certain types of physical handicap may be associated with psychiatric problems; for example, epilepsy (63, 380) and deafness (91). In some areas, special schemes may be required to bring psychiatric care to sections of the community which normally receive too little attention: underprivileged minority groups, people of low socioeconomic status, and those in rural areas with inadequate local facilities. In all these instances, prevalence surveys can be helpful simply by acting as a gauge of the current needs of the population. Of greater importance for long-term planning, however, are studies of the *trends* in disease incidence which can act as guides to probable future demand.

CHANGING TRENDS IN PSYCHIATRIC MORBIDITY

Much of the research on this subject has served to show that trends suggested by the official statistics were artefacts due to changes either in the provision and utilization of services, or in methods of recording and data-analysis (94, 379). Thus, Dayton (90) concluded that the increase in mental hospital beds in Massachusetts, between 1917 and 1933, corresponded to an increasing duration of hospital stay rather than to a rise in admissions. Goldhammer and Marshall, in their well-known study of Massachusetts hospital statistics over a century (157), found a progressive increase of mental disorder among the elderly, but no evidence of any real increase in the young and middle-aged groups. Mental hospital facilities in the area concerned had probably been adequate throughout the period; nevertheless, the possibility remained that attitudes had changed in a way which made people less willing to care for the elderly infirm at home and more ready to have them admitted to institutions.

More recently, there has been a conspicuous trend towards shorter duration of hospital stay: a development which seems to have antedated the appearance of tranquillising drugs in the 1950s. Shepherd, comparing cohorts of patients admitted to an English county mental hospital in 1931-33 and in 1945-47 (420), found a shorter length of stay and a higher discharge rate for the latter group. Hospitals which had pursued a liberal policy of early discharge and rehabilitation before the advent of tranquillisers were less dramatically affected than those which had previously been conservative in their policies (424).

Evidence of real change in the inception and prevalence of mental abnormality, rather than in the use of hospital services, is extremely hard to come by; it is, in fact, limited to situations where a survey of a given population has been replicated on one or more occasions after an interval of at least a generation. The outstanding example is that of the trend of intelligence among Scottish schoolchildren (418). The possibility of a falling national intelligence level due to differential fertility had been for many years a cause of concern to geneticists and others. A survey of all Scottish children born in 1921, undertaken in their eleventh year, afforded an opportunity to investigate the matter. In 1947, the survey was replicated, this time on children born in 1936. The same research design and method—notably the same group intelligence test—was used in both surveys. No significant change was found in the mean scores and, although certain difficulties interfered with a detailed comparison of the score-distribution (172), the findings indicated at least a possibility that the proportion of very low scores had actually diminished over the fifteen-year interval. It is a remarkable fact that the Scottish study remains virtually unique; and even here the investigation was in one sense retrospective, since the initial survey had not been planned as part of a time-trend enquiry.

Measurement of intelligence is sufficiently reliable to allow of direct comparison between the findings of different surveys even where the techniques have not been replicated. Goodman and Tizard, for example, compared their survey of mental retardation among schoolchildren in Middlesex, England (159), with the results of Lewis' investigation thirty years earlier (278). They found that, in the seven to 14 age-range, the rate for severe subnormality had fallen from 3.88 to 3.45 per thousand. That this had occurred while the prevalence of mongolism was rising sharply, because of increasing survival rates, strongly suggested a decline in the prevalence of severe subnormality, other than mongolism. Kushlick obtained similar results from a survey of defective children in an English rural area (257); he considered, however, that Lewis' figures may have been misleading because of the inclusion of a number of children without brain-damage, who were in truth of the "subcultural" type of retardation and who would not have been classified as mentally defective in more modern surveys.

The argument is far from academic, since on it to some extent hinges the estimation of future needs for medical and educational services. In most countries today, such services for the mentally retarded are grossly inadequate; if we can expect a continuing rise in the numbers of the handicapped, because of wider use of antibiotics and other modern forms of treatment, the strain on existing facilities must become insupportable. On the other hand, it is to be hoped that a rising standard of obstetric and neonatal care will begin to be reflected in a reduction of para-natal brain damage. Whatever trends emerge will require careful monitoring.

The hazards of trying to predict future trends are well shown by the controversy over psychiatric bed requirements for England and Wales. The fall in bed-occupancy which began unexpectedly in the 1950s, whether consequent on the introduction of tranquillising drugs or stemming from other causes, had implications for the planning of future mental health services. Tooth and Brooke (455) undertook a statistical analysis based partly on the rate of attrition of the existing long-stay population, partly on the projected build-up of a new generation of chronic patients not amenable to modern treatment methods. They came to the conclusion that by 1975 the bed-requirement would stabilize at about 1.8 per thousand population, compared with the 1959 rate of 3.3 per thousand, a drop of some 60,000 in the total number of beds for the country. This prediction was accepted by a government Hospital Plan, which translated prediction into policy by declaring that "A ratio of 1.8 beds per 1,000 population has therefore been taken as the probable limit of requirements by 1975" (328).

Critics were not slow to point out the risks inherent in extrapolating from a short-term trend, particularly in a situation where the number of hospital *admissions,* as distinct from the bed-occupancy, was continuing to rise steadily. The fallacy whereby a statistical prediction becomes transmuted first into a goal, and thence into official policy, without any recognition of the underlying dynamics of the situation, received a good deal of acerbic comment:

> Patients can be discharged, and beds can be emptied, by administrative decision: but, in the absence of some substantial and favourable

change in the situation, this can be achieved only at the cost of much hardship to patients and their families (160).

How far the official prediction will be wide of the mark is still not clear. By 1968, the bed-occupancy rate had fallen from 3.3 to 2.5 per thousand; in other words, just after half-time nearly half the expected drop had occurred. One must assume, however, a diminishing return on active rehabilitation policies; since when all the patients of relatively good prognosis have been discharged, there will remain a residue of chronic patients whose medical and social problems cannot be resolved. Case-register statistics have provided some support for this view, as in the Camberwell data illustrated by Figure 2.

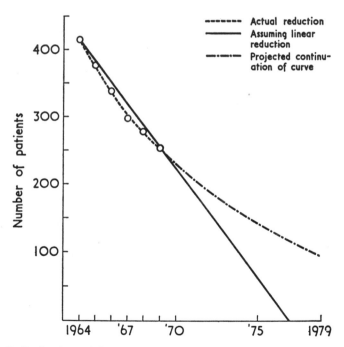

Figure 2. Reduction of long-stay population. Camberwell residents in hospital more than one year on 31 December 1964. Source: Hailey (178).

EVALUATION OF MENTAL HEALTH SERVICES

The controversy over psychiatric bed needs for England and Wales provides an illustration of one kind of confusion which can arise when operational research is not clearly distinguished from the *evaluation* of services. Evaluative studies derive much of their basic information from the statistics of service-utilization; but such data are of little significance unless they can be related to clearly defined aims and objectives. It is axiomatic that any such definitions must be couched at least partially in terms of the *needs* of patients and their families, and of sick persons in the community who are not in contact with the existing services. Wing *et al.* (477) have formulated the criteria for evaluation as a series of questions:

1. How many and what kinds of individuals are in contact with existing services?
2. What are their needs and those of their relatives? That is, what are their symptoms and disabilities, both primary and secondary, and what burdens are placed upon relatives and the rest of the community?
3. Are the services at present provided meeting these needs?
4. How many others, not in touch with existing services, also have needs and are they different from the needs of patients who do see psychiatrists?
5. What new services, or modifications to existing services, are likely to cater for unmet needs?
6. When innovations are introduced, do they in fact meet these needs?

In the past, medical administrators have placed little weight on research findings when planning the growth and development of services. Very little systematic research was undertaken into the working of psychiatric services until quite recently. As long as the provision of custodial care remained the main plank in these services, little need for planning was evident, especially since, in most industrial nations, one legacy of the nineteenth century had been a bountiful supply of asylum buildings. The modern emphasis on active treatment, extramural facilities and community care has changed this situation radically: the need for forward planning has become imperative and, in consequence, evaluative studies have begun to proliferate.

Methods of evaluating mental health services have been reviewed by Brandon and Gruenberg (36), who point out that hospital admission and discharge statistics alone are of limited value because they can so easily be manipulated. For example, a patient who had had only one or two brief spells outside hospital over a period of years would not be classed as a chronic case if the operational definition stipulated continuous in-patient care. Social indices such as unemployment, crime and divorce rates are also unsatisfactory, being subject to a variety of environmental factors. Realistic evaluation demands definition in three areas: first, the service must be described; secondly, its objectives must be firmly stated; thirdly, the population it serves must be demarcated. Ideally, evaluative measures should be applied simultaneously to a comparable population not receiving the service in question. Because of the difficulty of delineating comparable populations, an alternative method sometimes employed is to compare measures of the same population before and during the operation of a service: that is, to use the population as its own control.

These principles were applied by Gruenberg to the evaluation of the Dutchess County Project, New York State, which aimed at providing an integrated service for psychiatric patients from a defined catchment area. From its inception in 1960, the stated aim was to reduce the disability associated with psychotic illness, according to the following hypothesis:

> Chronic hospitalization and disability can be reduced by supplying the population with a comprehensive psychiatric service based upon a small, community-oriented, open public mental hospital so organized that there is a maximum of continuity of care over both in-patient and out-patient phases of treatment (208).

Community-based services were thus envisaged not merely as more humane than the traditional institutional care, but also as therapeutically more effective. It was hoped, indeed, that they would obviate the harmful features of institutional life, while at the same time increasing public tolerance of the mentally ill. Situated within the precincts of the Hudson River State Hospital, the unit retained full clinical autonomy; evaluation was undertaken by a team from Columbia University and the Milbank Memorial Fund (175).

Clinicians concerned with the day-to-day work of the unit were convinced of the benefits accruing from clinical autonomy, improved channels of communication and the close liaison with community services which the experiment provided. Such benefits, though apparent to the people most directly concerned, may be extremely difficult to measure and to demonstrate, partly because they concern intangibles. In the last analysis, a medical service must be evaluated principally in terms of its overall effect on the symptoms and functional impairment of patients.

Gruenberg (173) considered that, in relation to the psychoses, change could be effected most readily in such "behavioural distortions" as disorganized behaviour, combativeness, suicidal tendencies, deterioration and vegetable existence. In seeking a valid measure of the effectiveness of the service, he set up a construct of "Social Breakdown Syndrome" (SBS), defined as consisting of the secondary complications of psychotic illness which are related to environmental factors and so potentially preventable. The components of this syndrome were listed as withdrawal, self-neglect, dangerous behaviour, shouting, self-harm, failure to work and failure to enjoy recreation. It is thus not a medical syndrome in the true sense, but corresponds roughly to what Wing and other British workers have called "institutionalism" or the "secondary handicaps" of psychotic illness (472). In fact, as both Gruenberg and Wing have made clear, such handicaps are not restricted to mental hospital patients, but occur to some extent among psychotic persons in the community. Nonetheless, their appearance is favoured by the environment of the "total institution" (145).

An instrument for case-identification was developed, using well-defined behavioural criteria (174). A 10 percent sample of all patients in the population concerned, who had been in mental institutions at some time since 1955, was interviewed and rated on the basis of behaviour during the preceding seven days: the survey entailed assessment both of patients in hospital and of ex-patients in the community. The point -prevalence of severe chronic Social Breakdown Syndrome determined in this way was 50 per 100,000 of the adult population at the end of 1962. Its prevalence before the development of the community-centred service was thought (on the basis of a retrospective manipulation of the data) to have been twice as high. Although, on this evidence, the possibility of a general secular trend could not be ignored, the investigators concluded that "there seems to be good reason to believe that the comprehensive integrated mental health services, as rendered by the Dutchess County Unit, have prevented chronic social breakdown syndrome" (175) .

A more authoritative evaluation of a mental hospital service was that conducted in three English hospitals by the Medical Research Council (475) . This group of studies began as an "experiment of opportunity" when, in 1960, the appointment of a new medical superintendent at Severalls Hospital, Essex, inaugurated a vigorous programme of rehabilitation and administrative reform. This change of policy, in a hospital not previously noted for its active or progressive regime, afforded a chance of measuring the effects on the chronic institutional population: the relation between hospital environment and clinical symptoms postulated by Belknap (22) , Goffman (145) and others could now be put to a scientific test.

The research design consisted in essence of an initial comparative survey of the clinical and social condition of long-stay patients at Severalls and at two of the most advanced English mental hospitals, followed by a longitudinal study in which changes in all three groups of patients could be monitored as the new administration policy at Severalls took effect. The two "control" hospitals, Netherne and Mapperley, were both well known for their programmes of social psychiatry and each was outstanding as an example of a particular approach to the problems of the chronic mental patient. At Netherne, the emphasis for some years had been on an active rehabilitation programme within the hospital (26, 129) ; whereas at Mapperley, efforts had focused on the development of an integrated area service with early discharge and after-care as the means of preventing institutionalism (297, 298).

In order to measure the relevant clinical and social variables, a number of scales had to be constructed and tested, notably a simple, reliable rating of schizophrenic symptoms (471). Once these instruments were available, it was possible to measure clinical and social change independently and this was done on comparable samples of long-stay female schizophrenic patients at the three hospitals.

The initial survey showed that the patients at Severalls were conspicuously more deteriorated than their counterparts at the other two hospitals, the differences not being accountable in terms of any selective process of admission or discharge. Moreover, when the three patient samples were grouped together, significant correlations were found between the ratings for a number of clinical and social variables. Table XVIII illustrates the more important findings.

TABLE XVIII

INTERCORRELATIONS BETWEEN CLINICAL AND SOCIAL RATINGS FOR FEMALE CHRONIC SCHIZOPHRENIC PATIENTS IN THE THREE MENTAL HOSPITALS

| | (n = 273) | | |
| | *Social Variables* | | |
Clinical Variables	*Outside Contact*	*Personal Possessions*	*Time Spent Unoccupied*
Social withdrawal	— 0.48	— 0.56	+ 0.63
Flatness of affect	— 0.47	— 0.55	+ 0.54
Poverty of speech	— 0.34	— 0.52	+ 0.46
Incoherence of speech	— 0.18	— 0.13	+ 0.21
Coherently expressed delusions	+ 0.14	+ 0.30	+ 0.25
Socially embarrassing behaviour	— 0.20	— 0.21	+ 0.25

Source: Wing and Brown (475).

Over the ensuing years, the social environment of the Severalls patients showed a marked, steady upgrading, with a corresponding improvement in their clinical state. At the same time, unforeseen changes at the "control" hospitals led to a decline in the social ratings of the Mapperley patients after 1962, and of the Netherne patients after 1964. In both instances, a corresponding decline was found in the clinical condition of the patients. Within each hospital, a positive correlation was found between social and clinical scores over the follow-up period, the closest association being that between the level of planned occupation and recreational activities on the one hand, and the extent of patients' withdrawal on the other. Figure 3 illustrates the pattern for selected ratings.

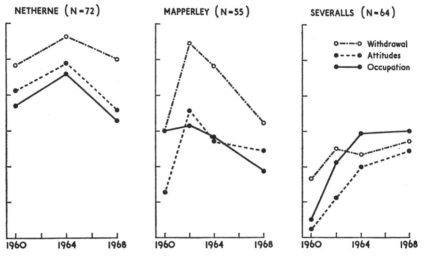

Figure 3. Three measures of clinical and social conditions of schizophrenic patients in three mental hospitals, 1960-1968. Source: Wing and Brown (475).

These findings, although open to some criticism, provide a striking example of the scientific evaluation of a psychiatric hospital service. In so doing, they help to modify the orthodox model of schizophrenia, confirming that the familiar clinical picture of the chronic, deteriorated patient is in some measure the result of an impoverished social environment.

Evaluation of community services is more difficult, because of the problems of monitoring clinical change and identifying all the variables by which it may be influenced. Nevertheless, a number of studies in recent years have contributed to our knowledge of this field and pointed the way to more substantial achievements in future.

In the field of mental retardation, Tizard was able to demonstrate the advantage of small residential units over the large institution (454). A sample of severely subnormal children from the Fountain Hospital, London, was transferred to Brooklands, a small house standing in its own grounds some miles out in the countryside. Run on the lines of a nursery school, with family groups and housemothers, Brooklands was intended to provide a secure but stimulating social environment. The experimental group was matched with a clinically similar control group of children who remained in the parent institution, and repeated intelligence testing was carried out on both groups. A marked and significant rise occurred in the verbal mental age of the Brooklands children as compared with the controls, whereas no significant differences were found in the non-verbal intelligence scores. The findings are illustrated by Figure 4.

Tizard's conclusion that such small residential units should be given an important place in future mental subnormality services has been taken up in the Wessex region of England, where a large-scale evaluative study is now being conducted (258).

The development of an English community service for mental illness has been studied in detail by a Medical Research Council team. This project grew out of the "Worthing Experiment" (57), which comprised the introduction of greatly extended out-patient and domiciliary facilities in the town of Worthing, Sussex. The primary objective was to reduce the rate of admission to Graylingwell Hospital, the area mental institution, where overcrowding had become a serious problem, as, indeed, it was in many British mental hospitals at that time.

Under the experimental scheme, no patient from Worthing was admitted to the mental hospital without first being seen in the community by a psychiatrist; previously, most admissions had come direct from general practitioners and mental welfare officers. Domiciliary screening by psychiatrists led to a 56 percent reduction in admissions during the first year of the experiment. Encouraged by this result, the local psychiatrists and administrators next introduced a similar scheme in the neighbouring town of Chichester; at the same time, day hospital facilities were developed within the curtilage of the mental hospital.

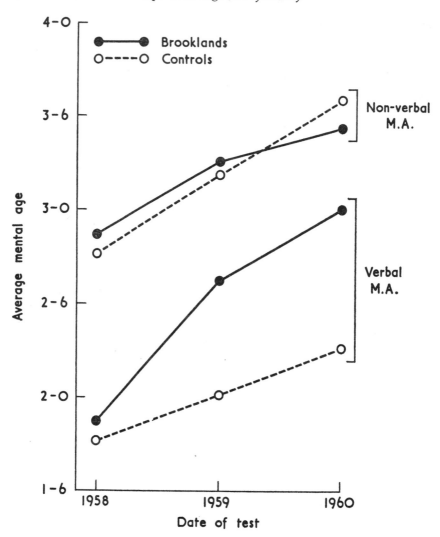

Figure 4. The Brooklands Experiment. Intelligence test results for experimental and control groups of mentally handicapped children. Source: Tizard (454).

More recently, the Medical Research Council team has conducted a series of evaluative studies in which the Chichester service has been compared with the more traditional hospital service for another cathedral town, Salisbury. Sainsbury and his colleagues (161, 162) have examined various aspects of the two services, in order to establish any differences in referral patterns, in clinical outcome, and in the effect on patients' families. Home interviews at the time of referral showed no difference between the two towns in the burden on patients' relatives. When a second assessment was made some weeks later, the traditional type of service at Salisbury appeared to be providing more relief to the families. This difference was concentrated among the relatively mild cases, the families of severely disturbed psychiatric patients being equally helped in the two populations.

On the basis of this research, it appears that community-centred services may well impose a heavier burden than the ordinary hospital-based service on the relatives of certain types of patient. The disparity, however, is less striking than might have been supposed, and has to be weighed against the advantages for the patient of avoiding mental hospital admission. Clearly, further longitudinal investigations will be required before the merits and demerits of community care can be adequately assessed.

One important aspect of the change-over to a community-based system is the possible effect on local suicide rates. Over a two-year period, the incidence of suicide in Chichester did not differ from that in Salisbury, the respective rates being 7.4 and 7.2 per 1,000 patients in contact with the services. A comparison of local suicide statistics before and after the introduction of the experimental scheme at Chichester (462) provided no evidence that the policy of treating patients in the community had increased their risk of self-harm.

Since 1963, suicide rates in Great Britain have been falling steadily. No adequate explanation has been given for this trend, which runs counter to those for the utilization of psychiatric services and for various indices of social pathology. Two plausible theories relate the fall to the advent of tricyclic antidepressant drugs in the late 1950s and to the more recent introduction of non-toxic natural gas as a domestic fuel. Another possible contributory factor has been the growth of Samaritan schemes in many British cities (19).

The Samaritan movement, first established in Britain in 1953, aims at encouraging potentially suicidal persons to make telephone contact with a voluntary helping service which operates on a 24-hour emergency basis (124). Doubts have been expressed as to whether this scheme helps the truly suicidal individual. Certainly, when compared with those who commit suicide, Samaritan clients as a whole show a very different profile: on average they are younger, more often female and more often of married status. It can be conjectured that they include a high proportion of persons who are not at high risk for suicide, but who tend to seek help and attention from any available social agency. On the other hand, a survey of six English towns (20) showed that those who contacted the Samaritans had a suicide rate of 357 per million in the ensuing year: a rate over twice that for the parent population. To this extent, it appears that the Samaritans are dealing with a suicide-prone clientele.

The question remains as to whether Samaritan schemes have any effect on local suicide rates. As a first step towards answering this question, Bagley undertook an ecological survey (12). Fifteen towns in England and Wales were selected, in which Samaritan groups had been operating for at least two years prior to the most recent suicide statistics. Control towns were selected by means of a systematic procedure using available social data on British towns (333). The average suicide rates for the Samaritan towns before and after the instigation of Samaritan schemes were compared with those for the control towns during the same periods of time. In view of the unexpected finding that this group of control towns had experienced an average rise of 19 percent in suicide rates during the survey period, a second set of control towns was drawn, closely matching the Samaritan towns in age, sex and social class distribution. The results of the two sets of comparisons are summarized in Table XIX.

From these findings, Bagley concluded that Samaritan schemes had been associated with a relative decline in suicide-risk in those towns where they had operated, so that even where the rates showed an absolute increase, this was smaller than in the corresponding control towns. The association could not be claimed as

TABLE XIX
SUICIDE RATES PER 100,000 POPULATION IN A GROUP OF BRITISH
TOWNS WITH SAMARITAN SCHEMES AND IN MATCHED CONTROL
TOWNS

	Samaritan Towns	*First Control Group*	*Second Control Group*
Average rate before Samaritan scheme	13.03	12.56	13.05
Average rate after Samaritan scheme	12.27	15.05	14.00
Overall percentage change	− 5.84	+ 19.84 ($p < 0.01$)	+ 7.23 ($p < 0.05$)

Source: Bagley (12).

causal, since for any town the same underlying social factors might have been responsible both for the setting-up of a Samaritan scheme and for a subsequent reduction in the suicide rate. Nevertheless, an association has been demonstrated and the case for more direct evaluative studies is unarguable.

The foregoing examples illustrate the scope for epidemiology in the evaluation both of existing mental health services and of planned programmes of change in these services. Involvement in this sphere is not without its drawbacks for the medical investigator. Being understandably keen that his findings and recommendations should be given their due weight in the planning of services, he can appreciate the merits of any system which will promote direct interchange between research groups and administrators. At the same time, he values greatly his position as an independent scientific worker who can pursue his own course without regard to the changing winds of bureaucratic concern. Between these conflicting interests, a compromise has to be effected. If in the short term research findings continue to exercise little influence on policy decisions, those that stand the test of time will serve ultimately to produce a new climate of opinion, not least by the way in which they affect the thinking of practising clinicians.

Chapter Four

USES OF EPIDEMIOLOGY
II. CLINICAL APPLICATIONS

T HE VALUE of epidemiological research has been much more widely recognized in the public health field, where its importance for prevention is well understood, than in clinical medicine, largely, no doubt, because of the clinician's inevitable preoccupation with individual patients. Nevertheless, epidemiology has direct relevance for medical practice, in two ways. First, any physician may use a basically epidemiological approach in seeking the origin and mode of transmission of disease among his patients. Secondly, every diagnosis relies upon actuarial data, since it consists in essence of a statement of probability about the aetiology, pathology, course and outcome of disease, and its response to treatment. Clinical thinking is thus constantly being influenced by morbidity statistics in general and by survey findings in particular. In short, the physician in his everyday practice makes use both of clinical and of statistical epidemiology.

CLINICAL EPIDEMIOLOGY

The role of the clinical epidemiologist, says Paul,

> . . . is like that of a detective visiting the scene of the crime. He starts with the examination of a sick individual and cautiously branches out into the setting where that individual became ill and where the patient may also become ill again. In this respect, the *clinical* epidemiologist stands in relation to the *statistical* epidemiologist perhaps as a physician does to a health officer. The statistician may validate his analyses by increasing the number of observations, whereas the clinician has the opportunity of improving the accuracy of a limited number of observations by intimate study and exacting measurements, This restriction of the size of the groups with which the clinical epidemiologist deals is certainly not essential, but it rests on the fact that clinical talents, carried out within the framework of an intimate doctor-patient relationship, cannot be readily applied wholesale, without the risk of their being spread too thinly to be effective (364) .

As an instance of this type of detective work, Paul cites the century-old story of Zenker and trichinosis. Having found the parasites of trichinae in the body of a young woman who had died shortly after admission to hospital, Zenker visited the inn where she had been employed as a maidservant, to discover that the landlord and his wife had been taken ill at about the same time. Numerous encapsulated trichinae were found in meat from a hog slaughtered two weeks earlier; moreover, the butcher who had killed the animal had also become sick. Zenker concluded that all these illnesses had probably resulted from the consumption of trichinous pork.

In this instance, the trail led back from the autopsy room to the patient's home and local community; at other times, the mode of transmission has been discovered without recourse to hospital investigation. A family physician with an interest in the "natural history" of disease (414) may plot the spread of an epidemic among his patients with the aid of no other tools than a pocketbook and pencil. Thus it was that William Pickles, for many years a general practitioner in the Yorkshire dales, plotted the incubation periods and patterns of spread of acute infectious fevers (378).

Mental disorders are not usually thought of as communicable; nevertheless, fundamentally similar methods are used in psychiatry. Epidemics of mental disorder still occur in our society, if less dramatically and on a smaller scale than in the Middle Ages. Local outbreaks can occasionally be ascribed to toxic substances. Such dangers arise in industry from the use of heavy metals and of organic compounds such as trichlorethylene (163, 434). They may also be due to naturally-occurring substances: an extraordinary epidemic of hallucinosis in a French village has been attributed to ergot poisoning from the consumption of infected rye (132). This well-documented episode has led to the suggestion that some of the so-called "hysterical" epidemics of former times may have had a similar basis.

More frequently, the transmitting agent appears to be suggestion or imitation, so that the epidemic is best regarded as a large-scale example of "socially-shared psychopathology" (171). Investigation of an acute epidemic in a girls' school (335) pointed strongly to a psychological rather than an infectious cause, most of the symptoms being attributable to overbreathing and the somatic correlates of anxiety. No infectious agent was isolated and all laboratory investigations were negative. The condition had developed first among the older girls and spread thence to the younger age-groups, whose members were less severely affected. The outbreak followed a local outbreak of poliomyelitis which had been widely publicized; moreover, it appeared to have been triggered off by a school church-parade during which some children had fainted. Comparison with an acute infectious epidemic at another school showed that the two types of outbreak could be clearly differentiated by their mode of onset and spread (318).

More recently, a retrospective study of an acute epidemic which led to the temporary closure of a London teaching hospital has raised the suspicion that this perplexing episode may also have been largely or entirely psychogenic (316). The epidemic developed with explosive rapidity during the summer of 1955. By the end of the first month, more than 100 cases had been reported; the hospital had to be closed and remained out of action for three months. The illness began with non-specific prodromal symptoms and in about three-quarters of all cases progressed to a stage of apparent central nervous involvement lasting for weeks or even months. Symptoms at this stage included slight pyrexia, vertigo, blurred vision or diplopia, motor weaknesses and sensory disturbance, especially parasthesiae and spontaneous pain. In some instances, "fits" were recorded, although none seem to have been definitely epileptic.

The diagnosis gave rise to much difficulty, the signs and symptoms failing to conform to any of the more obvious possibilities. Laboratory investigations were all negative and, in particular, all cerebrospinal fluid examined was normal. Most observers considered that a viral infection of the central nervous system had been responsible, and the name "benign myalgic encephalomyelitis" was proposed for this and a number of similar outbreaks (260). Thereafter, this diagnostic label was attached to many sporadic cases as well as to local epidemics.

In their reappraisal (316), McEvedy and Beard underlined a number of points which seemed to them to argue strongly against an infective origin. First, the outbreak had been virtually confined to the nursing staff of the hospital, and among them largely to females: the male-female ratio was variously estimated as 1:4 and (using more stringent case-criteria) as 1:13. Secondly, serological tests did not confirm the presence of viral infection. Thirdly, all observers agreed that the intense malaise and subjective symptoms—notably pain—were disproportionate to the objective clinical signs. Fourth, the disturbance of sensation seemed often to have conformed to the "glove-and-stocking" distribution traditionally associated with hysteria. Finally, as Table XX demon-

TABLE XX

INCIDENCE OF VARIOUS SYMPTOMS IN THE ROYAL FREE HOSPITAL
EPIDEMIC AND AMONG SCHOOLGIRLS INVOLVED IN A HYSTERICAL
EPIDEMIC

Incidence of Symptoms (Prodromal) Royal Free Hospital Epidemic		Incidence of Equivalent Symptoms Girls' School Epidemic	
	%		%
Headache	77	Headache	59
Sore throat	63	No equivalent	
Malaise	62)	General weakness	40
Lassitude	51)		
Vertigo	47)	Dizziness	63
Dizziness	33)		
Nausea	40	Nausea	44
Pains in limbs	46	No equivalent	
Pain in back	32)	Pain in back or abdomen	44
Pain in abdomen	14)		
Stiff neck	32	Pain in chest or neck	18
Depression	19	Feeling of panic	25
Vomiting	12	Vomiting	10
Diplopia, tinnitus, diarrhoea	10		

Source: McEvedy and Beard (316).

strates, the pattern of prodromal symptoms was similar to that which McEvedy had found among hysterical schoolgirls.

On the strength of their findings, and having reviewed 15 recorded outbreaks of "benign myalgic encephalomyelitis," the investigators suggested that this label should be dropped:

As there seems to be a total lack of objective evidence in support of the view that in cases of benign myalgic encephalomyelitis the brain and spinal cord are the site of an infective, inflammatory disease process, we would suggest that the name be discarded. Even if the view that the symptoms are hysterical is not accepted, it would seem prudent to shorten it to "benign myalgia." Our own inclination is for 'myalgia nervosa' on the analogy of "anorexia nervosa." This could serve both for the epidemic illness and for any isolated cases of functional disorder which conform to the same clinical picture (317).

A somewhat different problem which may confront the psychiatrist is that of tracing the source of a local outbreak whose aetiology is well established. This kind of problem has been called "community diagnosis" (331) in contradistinction to patient diagnosis. An example is provided by the recent rapid increase of heroin abuse in Great Britain, which has presented medical workers in some areas with a serious epidemic. Suspecting that the prevalence of addiction in one English town was much higher than the official estimates, two local psychiatrists undertook a screening survey of the young adult population (7). For this purpose, they employed five screening methods: (1) local probation officer reports; (2) local police reports; (3) a survey of hospital casualty department records for cases of drug overdosage; (4) a survey of hospital in-patient records for cases of jaundice among young patients; (5) the reports of known heroin users. Of these five methods, the last two proved most effective, yielding 20 and 46 confirmed cases, respectively.

The findings of this survey indicated a prevalence rate of 8.5 per 1,000 in the age-group 15 to 20, as against the official estimate of 1.4 per 1,000. The question remained as to how far the former, more realistic figure signified a new epidemic: a point which Alarcon (6) went on to investigate by a study of the spread of heroin abuse in the local population. By establishing for each case the approximate date of first injection and the identity of the initiator, he showed that the incidence of this condition had risen steeply following an initial latent period, and that the rise was attributable to direct person-to-person spread. In short, the pattern conformed to that usually regarded as characteristic of infectious epidemics. Two major transmission trees, each stemming from an initiator outside the town, accounted for no fewer than 48 confirmed cases. Figure 5 shows the main transmission

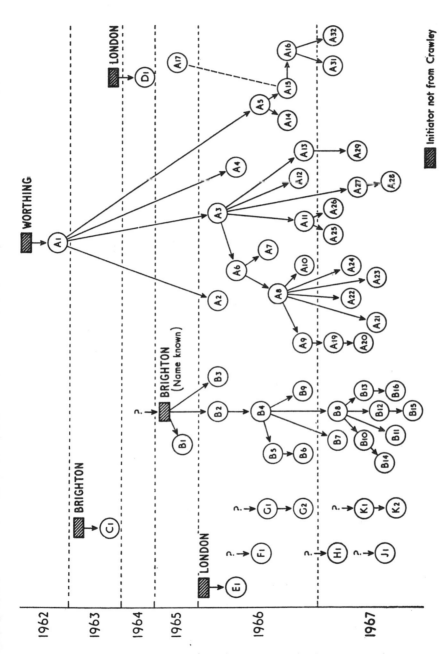

Figure 5. Transmission of heroin abuse in Crawley New Town. Source: Alarcon (6).

trees and the manner in which they produced an exponential increase of narcotic abuse.

In each of these studies, the investigators were concerned with the spread of a disease among the susceptible members of an institution or community. For the majority of mental disorders, which are endemic and widely distributed throughout the general population, this method of enquiry is inappropriate. There is, nonetheless, one aspect of the communication of mental abnormality in which psychiatrists have long retained a special interest, namely, spread within the nuclear family. The subject is complex, demanding investigation in its genetic, epidemiological, clinical and psycho-social aspects. A relatively simple approach adopted by some workers is the charting of family morbidity experience over a number of years, to test the possibility that illness episodes tend to occur in clusters.

Once again, the technique owes its origin to the study of infectious disease. Examination of family medical records revealed, for example, that the onset of poliomyelitis in some children could be related to undiagnosed episodes of headache, vomiting and malaise among their siblings. Dingle and his co-workers in Cleveland, Ohio, found wide differences in family rates of upper respiratory infection, and showed that they could be related to social factors (93). A study of families in Boston found that the incidence of streptococcal throat infections was related to the family experience of stressful events in the preceding weeks (325).

In studies of this kind, the transmission of specific disease agents could be assumed. At the same time, it was becoming apparent that family clustering of illness episodes was restricted neither to specific diagnoses nor to infectious disease as a whole. Kellner (229), reporting on the morbidity-experience of some 350 families over a two-year period, found a tendency for all kinds of ill-health to be grouped into family episodes. A typical example is shown in Figure 6, which summarizes the consultation records for a family of five people.

The family illness-experience on which this summary-chart is based can be adumbrated as follows:

12th June   Younger daughter ill, complaining of sore throat.

	1958												1959											
	1	2	3	4	5	6	7	8	9	10	11	12	1	2	3	4	5	6	7	8	9	10	11	12
Mother 35						x		x						x										
Daughter 7						x x x x x x x x							x											
Daughter 10						x x x x	x x		x															
Son 9							x x x						x x	x										
Father 38						x																x	x	

Figure 6. Family illness: a specimen case-record from general practice Source: Kellner (229)

Restless, flushed, temperature 104, pulse 120, enlarged neck glands. Mother anxious. Pyrexia persists for three days, then subsides; no residual symptoms.

15th June   Elder daughter and son both develop similar pyrexial illness.

16th June   Mother attends, complaining of long-standing pruritis vulvae (not previously reported). No cause found. Reassured.

20th June   Mother attends again; this time to ask for prescription for husband's haemorrhoids. Husband asked to attend but fails to do so.

Such a brief episode would be in no way remarkable were it not out of character for the family in question which, as the summary-chart shows, seldom troubled the doctor. While in this instance all the illnesses were minor, the episode showed some features common to much more serious "family epidemics." Although the main factor was an acute infectious condition, some of the consultations were for apparently unrelated, non-infective conditions. Chronic ailments came to light which had not been previously reported. The doctor was aware of an increase in hypochondriacal anxiety and health preoccupation in the mother, the central figure. Once the "epidemic" had subsided, no more mention was made of the non-infective conditions.

A family physician who is able to connect illnesses in this way can often make shrewd inferences about the underlying pathology and, indeed, the likely outcome of individual cases. No wider conclusions can be reached, unless care is taken to ensure that the observed patterns are truly representative. For this purpose, the illness-experience of a random sample of patients must be recorded systematically and defined in terms of the parent population, a point at which clinical epidemiology merges into statistical, and the function of the clinician gives way to that of the professional research worker.

COMPLETION OF THE CLINICAL PICTURE

Epidemiological research helps to ensure the proportional representation of all types and degrees of morbidity, and enables them to be seen against the background of subclinical and asymptomatic cases. This effect of putting clinical case-material into perspective—what Morris (331) has called "completing the clinical picture of disease"—represents one of the major contributions of the community survey to modern psychiatry.

The best-authenticated instances are drawn from the field of mental retardation. Since the time of Francis Galton, psychologists have been concerned to chart the relation of mental deficiency to normal intelligence, through the wide range of normal variation. A well-known example is the study of Stockholm children by Pearson and Jaederholm (366). A group of 300 children, excluded from ordinary schools on grounds of feeble-mindedness, was examined with a modified version of the Binet-Simon intelligence test. When a sample of the normal school population was also examined, it appeared that the distribution of intelligence scores for the two groups was continuous, with no indication of a natural boundary between the normal and the retarded children. Despite a fairly high correlation between test scores and clinical diagnosis, the ascertainment of mental deficiency by means of intelligence tests would have resulted in a subnormal group of somewhat different composition. (Fig. 7).

The blurring between normality and the cultural forms of mental retardation is now widely recognized. Even where defect states are associated with clearly defined constitutional abnormalities, the distinction between cases and normals is apt to be less clear-cut than hospital studies might suggest. Chromosome abnormalities, for example, are found in the general population, although less frequently than among mentally defective groups (372). Similarly, cases of phenylketonuria with measured intelligence in the normal range have been reported (10).

Perhaps the most striking instances of this function of epidemiology are those which have appeared as by-products of large-scale military conscription in the two world wars. In the words of Burt:

> It was perhaps the First World War that most effectively brought home to the medical world the artificiality of the distinction between the normal mind on the one hand and its abnormal conditions on the other. The application of intelligence tests to nearly two million

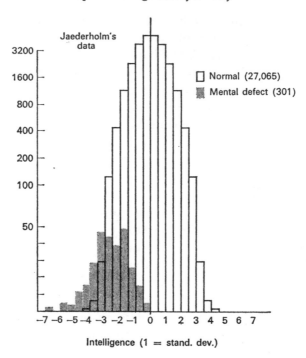

Figure 7. Distribution of intelligence among normal schoolchildren and mentally defective children in Stockholm. Source: Pearson and Jaederholm (366).

Americans led to the startling conclusion that nearly 40 per cent of the population had a mental age below the level then currently accepted as marking off the mentally defective (56).

Although more realistic standards were applied in the Second World War, the results of mass testing suggested the need for a further revision of standards. In the United States, for example, no fewer than 10 million men completed the Army General Classification Test, which had been validated as carefully as most such instruments. The distribution of scores did not correspond closely to a Gaussian curve, but showed some flattening and skewing, with fewer than expected numbers in the highest grade and more than expected in the lower grades. The observed and expected distributions are shown in Table XXI.

TABLE XXI
OBSERVED AND EXPECTED DISTRIBUTION OF SCORES, U.S. ARMY
GENERAL CLASSIFICATION TEST, SECOND WORLD WAR

Grade	Test Score	Observed Frequency	Expected Frequency
I	130 & over	5.8	7
II	110–130	26.2	24
III	90–110	30.7	38
IV	70–90	28.5	24
V	Below 70	8.8	7

Source: Bingham (27).

Initially, all men scoring less than 70 were graded as dullards, but in 1943 the threshold was lowered to a score of 60 because of the increasing demand for troops. The ability of many of these men to perform useful duties in wartime underlines the waste of human potential under ordinary peacetime conditions, and the extent to which definitions of feeble-mindedness are socially determined.

Epidemiological surveys have had less effect on clinical perspective in the field of mental illness, but here too they are gaining in importance. Three examples will serve to illustrate the trend. First, cross-cultural surveys are beginning to modify our thinking about the fundamental, biological aspects of mental illness. Exotic syndromes such as amok, latah, witigo, koro and Arctic hysteria are each peculiar to certain cultures (485). The major syndromes familiar to Western society have been found in all parts of the world, but vary in their clinical manifestations according to the prevailing culture. Catatonic rigidity, stereotypy and negativism are relatively frequent among Indian schizophrenic patients; withdrawal and passivity among those in preliterate African tribes (341). Ideas of guilt, self-reproach and suicide are reported to be less common among depressed patients in primitive societies than among those in the West (340). The course of the illness may also be determined to some extent by cultural factors: among indigenous tropical peoples, for example, schizophrenia appears to carry a more favourable prognosis than in Western society (339).

The second illustration is taken from child psychiatry. Most of the conduct and habit disorders seen in children are not intrinsically abnormal, but rather exaggerations or prolongations of normal behaviour patterns. Our notions of what is morbid in childhood behaviour have been profoundly influenced by the selective processes leading to psychiatric consultation and diagnosis, a point on which Kanner (222) has remarked:

> This selectiveness, in the absence of "normal controls," has often resulted in a tendency to attribute to single behaviour items an exaggerated "seriousness" with regard to their intrinsic psychopathological significance . . . in clinical statistics, those same symptoms, figuring among the traits found in the histories of "problem children," are apt to be given too prominent a place, far out of proportion to their role as everyday problems or near-problems of the everyday child.

To assess the importance of selective factors in psychiatric referral, we need information about the distribution in the child population of a wide range of behavioural items. The occurrence of any single item is of limited significance, deviance from the norm being related not only to questions of intensity, frequency and duration, but also to the age, sex and socio-cultural background of the child. In a survey of school-children in an English county (425), questions were put to the parents concerning the *frequency* of fifteen items of behaviour on an eight-point scale ranging from "never or less than once a year" to "every day or nearly every day". In addition, twenty-two triple-choice questions inquired into the *intensity* of behavioural items where this seemed more appropriate. An example of the first type of scale was frequency of complaints of stomach-pains. Figure 8 shows the resulting distribution for children of different ages from five to fifteen years; the increasing frequency for girls of from twelve years onwards is related to the onset of menstruation.

Data obtained in this way can be compared with information derived from the records of child psychiatrists or child guidance clinics. In the Buckinghamshire survey, deviance was measured by summing the scores for all those items present in less than 10 percent of a given age-group. When a group of fifty child guidance attenders was compared with fifty matched controls showing similar behavioural profiles, the index group received higher

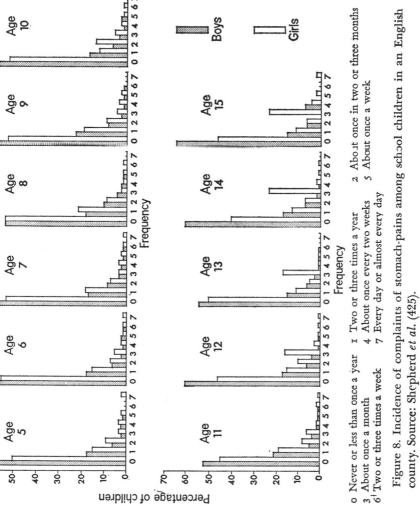

Figure 8. Incidence of complaints of stomach-pains among school children in an English county. Source: Shepherd *et al.* (425).

clinical severity ratings; nevertheless, it was held that this difference alone was insufficient to explain selective referral. Other factors, such as parental attitudes, must be considered as possibly important determinants of referral (Table XXII).

TABLE XXII

AVERAGE RATING-SCORE OF SEVERITY OF DISTURBANCE EXHIBITED BY CHILDREN ATTENDING CHILD GUIDANCE CLINICS AND A MATCHED CONTROL GROUP

Average Rating Score	Clinic Attenders	Nonclinic Group
1 "very mild"	1	1
2 "mild"	12	23
3 "moderate"	29	22
4 "severe"	8	4
	50	50

Source: Shepherd *et al.* (425).

These findings suggest that if the deviance scores of child guidance attenders were superimposed on the distribution for the whole sample of Buckinghamshire schoolchildren, they would fit into one tail of a Gaussian curve much as did the mentally retarded children in the Stockholm survey. The results of an American survey undertaken at about the same time presented a similar picture (266).

The third example is taken from adult psychiatry, where clinical perspectives are now being modified by the findings of community surveys. In Great Britain, data from general practice have thrown new light on the significance of hospital statistics. Table XXIII compares the diagnostic distribution of psychiatric in-patients and out-patients with that of a sample of psychiatric patients in a general practice population.

The differences shown in Table XXIII are understandable on the premise that psychoses are generally more severe and socially disabling conditions than neuroses, and hence tend to be selected more frequently both for psychiatric referral and for mental hospital admission. Nevertheless, these differences provide a useful reminder that the types of disorders which dominate hospital practice are not necessarily the most important for primary medical care.

TABLE XXIII

DISTRIBUTION OF THE MAIN PSYCHIATRIC CATEGORIES IN
HOSPITAL AND GENERAL PRACTICE

Diagnostic category	Mental Hospital First Admissions England and Wales 1957	Maudsley Hospital Out-patients 1956-1958	General Practice Survey Cases 1961-1962
	%	%	%
Psychoses	72.3	24.5	4.2
Neuroses	18.1	43.6	63.4
Character disorders	5.0	23.2	3.9
Miscellaneous	4.6	8.9	28.5
Total	100.0	100.0	100.0
Total no. of cases	48,266	6,752	2,049

Source: Cooper (75).

Similar considerations apply to the social and demographic distribution of psychiatric illness. A number of workers have reported a marked social class gradient in the prevalence of mental disorder, but these findings have been based on mental hospital data (116, 181), or on the records of all psychiatric agencies (204). General practice data are not highly reliable for social class; nonetheless, the complete absence of any social gradient in the general practice sample shown in Figure 9 provides a striking contrast with the great excess of low socio-economic status patients admitted to mental hospitals.

Other demographic characteristics which are subject to selective bias include age, sex, marital status, ethnic group and area of residence. It is possible that some of the features long regarded as characteristic of mental patients simply reflect the socio-cultural determinants of psychiatric referral and hospital admission. Without the help of epidemiological research, bias of this type could not be identified.

CLINICAL DIAGNOSIS AND CLASSIFICATION

The notion that psychiatric diagnosis is based on actuarial considerations is by no means new. Kraepelin's taxonomy was derived from observation of the symptom-groupings in large numbers of institutional patients, together with a careful study of the course

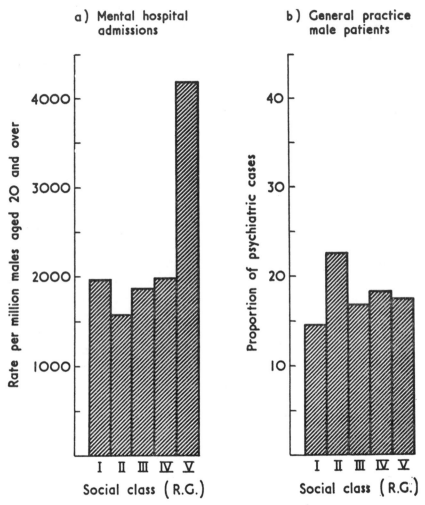

Figure 9. Social class distribution of psychiatric patients. (a) Mental hospital admissions, England and Wales, 1957. (b) Survey of 46 London general practices, 1961-1962. Source: Cooper (75).

and outcome of illness for each group (249, 353). So long as the aetiology and pathogenesis of many psychiatric disorders remain obscure, this approach provides the only practical basis for classification (205); as such it has been applied over the years to a wide range of conditions, from senile psychoses (402, 403) to the disorders of childhood (196, 395). The introduction of modern statistical techniques has done much to refine the Kraepelinian method without making any fundamental change.

So far, the epidemiologist's contribution to nosology has been small: partly because the necessary investigations have yet to be undertaken, partly because epidemiologists understandably prefer to use existing classifications, rather than to attempt any new delineation of syndromes. Indeed, the sharp differences found between the incidence and distribution of the main symptom groupings have been argued in support of the existing taxonomy (270). Cohort studies, for example, have provided support for the broad division into affective and schizophrenic psychoses.

Of relevance in this context is the survey of mental illness in London by Norris (347), who aimed at an objective appraisal of the course and outcome of treated mental illness, and the principal determinants thereof. All patients admitted to three mental hospitals and two observation wards, during the period 1947 to 49, were followed up to the end of 1951, any further hospital admissions being recorded. The resulting sample was large enough to permit of detailed analysis in terms of diagnosis, prognosis and various concomitant factors.

Taking as index the first admission diagnosis, which was obviously independent of outcome, the proportion of long-stay patients in the schizophrenic group was three times that in the manic-depressive group, while the latter in turn was three times that in the neurotic group. The findings for male patients between twenty and forty years are summarized in Table XXIV.

TABLE XXIV

MENTAL HOSPITAL ADMISSION AND RETENTION, BY DIAGNOSTIC CATEGORY: LONDON, 1947-1949

Admission Diagnosis	Percent of All Admissions	Percent of Each Category Remaining For One Year or More
Schizophrenia	54.5	44.1
Manic-depressive psychosis	23.4	15.8
Psychoneurosis	9.8	4.8
Organic psychosis	7.3	55.3
Character disorder	5.0	9.4

Source: Norris (347).

Norris concluded that the existing system had value both for administrative and for research purposes, and in particular that its prognostic significance was substantially confirmed. It may, of course, be objected that a survey which takes no account of patients outside hospital provides an inadequate basis for such a conclusion.

On occasion, prevalence surveys have helped to modify psychiatric taxonomy. The mental deficiency survey of England and Wales by Lewis (278) suggested that a relatively mild, culturally determined form of retardation could be distinguished from the more profound biological defects. A Swedish survey (442) which raised serious doubts about the existence of "Involutional Melancholia" as an entity, was partly responsible for the subsequent decline in use of that diagnosis. Conversely, a survey of an English county provided support for the belief that, at least so far as family incidence and social distribution are concerned, the syndrome of early child autism is quite distinct from schizophrenia (287).

THE PROGNOSIS FOR ESTABLISHED ILLNESS

While epidemiological research has thus at times affected diagnostic concepts, it has had a more marked influence on prognosis. Longitudinal studies in the community, though still few in number, have already provided the clinician with a number of valuable cross-bearings. As with prevalence surveys a generation earlier, the trend has been for cohort studies to focus initially on mental hospital patients and thence to extend to the community through consideration of discharged patients and their families. The research on institutionalism and schizophrenia, cited in the previous chapter, has been supplemented by studies of discharged patients in which their subsequent progress has been related to their type of living-group (43), their degree of emotional involvement with relatives (44), their occupational adjustment (330) and their experience of stressful events (42). Similar investigations have been conducted in the United States (127). It seems clear that the course and outcome of schizophrenic illness is heavily influenced by social factors, which have to be taken into account in assessing individual prognosis. These studies are important, not merely in the deterministic sense that they render prediction more accurate, but because they point to relatively specific social measures for improving the long-term outcome.

No comparable body of research has been undertaken on the course of the neuroses and character disorders. Greer and Cawley (168), having extensively reviewed the literature on this topic, concluded that "it is not possible to make legitimate generalisations about the prognosis of neurotic disorders from the published data." While their own thorough and detailed follow-up of a sample of psychiatric hospital in-patients overcame many of the defects of method evident in earlier studies, they emphasized the need for investigation of the milder types of neurotic illness which do not require hospital care.

A small beginning has been made by the study of patients under general medical care. In Great Britain, the general practitioner's registered patient list under the National Health Service constitutes a valuable sampling-frame. Longitudinal studies of neurotic illness in general practice populations (77, 186) suggest that the most important single prognostic factor is the current duration of symptoms; on this basis, a simple dichotomy can be established with, on the one hand, short-term situational reactions and, on the other, chronic neuroses having a low recovery-rate. Figure 10 illustrates a simple model for the changing distribution of neurotic illness in a general practice population.

These findings give some indication of the extent of chronic neurotic illness in the general population, and hence of its significance as a public health problem. A number of enquiries in recent years have begun to relate chronic neurosis to personality and physical constitution (184, 285), to physical ill-health (41, 103) and to social adjustment (76).

THE ASSESSMENT OF INDIVIDUAL MORBID RISK

Predictive factors, once identified, can be evaluated by means of anterospective enquiry, a technique which has been exploited to some purpose by criminologists (144, 306). Similarly, the clinical psychiatrist can be helped by longitudinal surveys to assess the risk of future morbidity in persons whose current mental state is

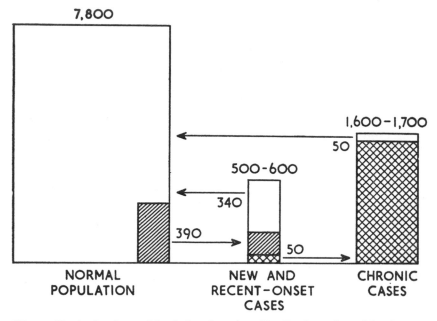

Figure 10. A simple model of the changing distribution of psychiatric morbidity during one year in a standard population of 10,000. Source: Harvey-Smith and Cooper (186).

normal or only mildly disturbed. This principle has been applied to the calculation of illness-expectancy among the relatives of patients with established mental disorder, the method of the "empirische Erbprognose" (426).

The same approach is equally relevant to the assessment of morbid risk for the patient himself in conditions where the occurrence of one or more previous attacks is held to influence the probability of future episodes. An obvious case in point is affective psychosis, since periodicity forms an integral part of the Kraepelinian view of manic-depression, and, indeed, long-term follow-up studies have tended to confirm this view (391). Unfortunately, the diagnostic reliability for this category has proved too poor for the findings of even the more intensive surveys to show any consistency. The expectancy rates shown in Table XXV, for example, are derived from some of the most careful and thorough studies, yet clearly the data are too unreliable to serve as a basis for clinical prediction.

TABLE XXV
EXPECTATION THROUGH LIFE OF AFFECTIVE DISORDER

Authors	Place of Survey	Expectancy Per 1,000 Births	
		Male	Female
Fremming (128)	Bornholm, Denmark	10.2	22.4
Larsson and			
Sjögren (268)	Sweden	9.0	12.0
Helgason (191)	Iceland	18.0	24.6
Ødegaard (350)	Norway	4.2	6.2
Norris (347)	London, England	8.0	14.4
Essen-Möller (111)	Sweden	17.0	28.0

Source: Rawnsley (385).

An application of greater practical importance is the assessment of suicide risk. Groups known to be at increased risk for suicide include patients suffering from manic-depressive illness (448), chronic alcoholics (238), and those persons who have already made at least one suicidal attempt.

Recent years have seen a marked increase in the numbers admitted to hospital because of self-injury which has not resulted in death: self-poisoning, in particular, has increased drastically. As a class, such patients differ in a number of respects from those who commit suicide: whereas the latter are still predominantly male, middle-aged or elderly, and living alone, the distribution for attempted suicide shows a preponderance of young people, women and those living in family groups. Nevertheless, attempted suicide patients as a whole constitute a high-risk group, and follow-up studies have shown that a significant proportion do subsequently kill themselves.

Tuckman and Youngman, in an attempt to identify the main risk factors (458), examined the records of some 1,100 adults who had come to the attention of the Philadelphia police as a result of suicidal attempts. The suicide rate for this sample over the next twelve months was 1,950 per 100,000, or 140 times the average rate for the city population. Eleven factors were identified as predictive

TABLE XXVI

SUICIDE RATES PER 1,000 POPULATION AMONG 1,112 ATTEMPTED SUICIDES, BY HIGH- AND LOW-RISK CATEGORIES OF RISK RELATED FACTORS

Factor	High-risk Category	Suicide Rate	Low-risk Category	Suicide Rate
Marital status	Separated, divorced, widowed	41.9	Single, married	12.4
Employment status*	Unemployed, retired	24.8	Employed†	16.3
Living arrangements	Alone	71.4	With others	11.1
Health	Poor (acute or chronic condition in the 6-month period preceding the attempt)	18.0	Good†	13.8
Mental condition	Nervous or mental disorder, mood or behavioural symptoms including alcoholism	17.6	Presumably normal, including brief situational reactions†	11.7
Method	Hanging, firearms, jumping, drowning	45.5	Cutting or piercing, gas or carbon monoxide, poison, combination of methods, other	13.1
Potential consequences of method	Likely to be fatal‡	31.5	Harmless, illness-producing	6.0
Police description of attempted suicide's condition	Unconscious, semiconscious	16.3	Presumably normal, disturbed, drinking, physically ill, other	13.0
Suicide note	Yes	22.5	No†	13.7
Previous attempt or threat	Yes	22.6	No†	13.3
Disposition	Admitted to psychiatric evaluation center	21.0	Discharged to self or relative; referred to family doctor, clergyman, or social agency; or other disposition	11.6

*Does not include housewives and students.
†Includes cases for which information on this factor was not given in the police report.
‡Several criteria used in estimating whether the method used was likely to be fatal.
Source: Tuckman and Youngman (458).

of repeat suicidal attempts and successful suicide. On the basis of their findings, which are summarized in Table XXVI, the investigators constructed a simple index of suicide risk which discriminated clearly between high- and low-risk individuals.

From the items listed in Table XXVI, together with those of age, sex and ethnic status, a fourteen-point scale of suicide risk was constructed. Using a total of four as the cut-off point, the suicide rate was estimated at 0.0 per 1,000 for the low-score group and 35.2 per 1,000 for the high-score group, a highly significant difference. Clearly, with larger samples and more detailed coverage the relative contribution of individual risk factors could be computed, and hence weighted scales could be derived with possibly greater predictive accuracy. Work along these lines is proceeding in a number of centres.

The investigation of high-risk groups, apart from its relevance for clinical prognosis, is a logical first stage in the identification of causal factors. By examining differences in the frequency of a given disorder as between different populations, or different sections of the same population, it is possible to test for associations between its rate of inception and various psychological, biological or social indices. It is to this search for causal factors, long regarded as the most important use of epidemiology, that we now turn.

Chapter Five

USES OF EPIDEMIOLOGY
III. THE SEARCH FOR CAUSES

IMPORTANT as are the administrative and clinical applications of epidemiology, there can be no doubt that its status as a major medical discipline has derived chiefly from the part which it has played in uncovering the causes of disease. In this context, the essential feature of the epidemiologist's method is his use of differential rates of incidence to test for associations between disease and the strength of various biological and environmental factors.

The achievements of epidemiology in the field of infectious disease are well known (481). More recently, the same approach has begun to make impressive contributions to the scientific study of non-infectious disease (38). Understandably, the results have been more dramatic where a single, specific causal agent could be identified. No doubt many such agents remain to be discovered; but medical investigators are being forced increasingly to postulate multifactorial causation, and to resign themselves to a gradual piecing together of the factors of disease. Nowhere does this hold more true than in psychiatry, where for at least a century the roles of host and environment have been accorded equal weight with those of the disease "agent" (170). In the early years of this century, the teaching of Adolf Meyer highlighted the importance of biographical "life-charts" for the understanding of individual mental pathology (324). Equally, for the study of mental illness in populations, consideration must be given to risk-factors which operate at any point of the life-span from conception to the onset of illness and beyond. For convenience, such risk-factors may be grouped together as those concomitant with the illness, those which operate immediately before its onset (precipitating factors), and those which operate over prolonged periods or at earlier phases of the life-span (predisposing factors).

CONCOMITANT FACTORS

The identification of biological and social concomitants of mental disorder represents a basic stage of aetiological research in psychiatry. This approach has been widely employed because it lends itself to investigation by prevalence surveys, the most readily practicable type of population study. Most enquiries have focussed on the demography and ecology of mental illness, looking for possible associations with age, sex, marital status, social class, ethnic status, religious persuasion and area of residence. From the extensive literature, two examples will suffice: the social class distribution in schizophrenia, and the association between physical and mental illness.

Social Class and Schizophrenia

Faris and Dunham (116), in the first major ecological study of mental disorder in an urban area, computed rates for the principal diagnostic categories in Chicago from 1922 to 1931, taking mental hospital admission as their case-criterion. They found the highest incidence of schizophrenia, as of alcoholic psychosis and neurosyphilis, in the poor, low-class central area of the city, the "necrotic hub" of Chicago, characterized by social deterioration and high mobility. Conversely, the lowest rates were found in the affluent middle-class suburbs. Possible sources of bias—notably selective hospital admission and the high mobility of population in the central areas—were considered by the investigators, but thought unlikely to explain the very big differences in incidence.

Two principal hypotheses were put forward to explain the ecological pattern. First, persons in the lower social groups and in the central areas might be subjected to increased social and economic stresses, which could be causally related to schizophrenia: this view became known as the *breeder* hypothesis. Secondly, the *drift* hypothesis suggested that those persons who develop schizophrenia have suffered from some prepsychotic abnormality or inadequacy of personality which has caused them to take progressively less responsible and remunerative work, and hence to sink in the social scale before the onset of frank psychotic symptoms.

Faris and Dunham were doubtful of the part played by downward social drift. While no decisive evidence could be adduced from their survey, the broadly comparable age-distributions of schizophrenia in different parts of the city argued against the drift hypothesis, which would lead one to predict a concentration of older, more chronic cases in the central areas. They concluded that the evidence favoured the "breeder" hypothesis:

> In these most disorganised sections of the city, and indeed of our whole civilization, many persons are unable to derive sufficient mental nourishment from the normal social sources to achieve a satisfactory conventional organization of their world. The result may be a lack of any organization at all, resulting in confused, frustrated and chaotic personality; or it may be a complex but unconventional original organization. In either case, there is a serious divergence from the conventional organization which makes communication and understanding impossible and, for that matter, makes any form of co-operation difficult. It is just this type of unintelligible behaviour which becomes recognized as mental disorder (116).

The skewed distribution of schizophrenia reported by Faris and Dunham was subsequently confirmed for nine American cities (65). Other workers found that the pattern varied according to the type of city: in a "political" as opposed to a commercial and industrial urban structure, the incidence of mental disorder was more closely related to ward rental values than to the density of population (23). In Bristol, England, Hare found a distribution broadly similar to that in Chicago, but because Bristol had no "necrotic hub," the social correlates of schizophrenia differed from those for the American city (182). A high incidence occurred in the "good" central area as well as in the poor rooming-house districts; the peripheral areas, where schizophrenia was least often found, were not in the main middle-class residential suburbs, but public housing developments.

The argument was taken a stage further by a study of male schizophrenic patients in Worcester, Massachusetts, (138), which showed a distribution similar to that in Chicago and other cities. When, however, the patients were divided into those who had been living alone and those admitted from their family homes, the characteristic ecological pattern was confined to the former group, a finding which suggested that the high incidence areas were breeding grounds only insofar as they encouraged or exacerbated social isolation.

Support for this hypothesis came from the survey by Hare (183), who reported that the differences in ward rates for Bristol were due chiefly to patients living alone or away from their families; those admitted from family households were randomly distributed throughout the city. Because the local ecological pattern did not fit the "drift" hypothesis in its original form, Hare proposed that it should be modified into a "segregation" hypothesis, which need not imply downward social mobility. What to his mind characterized the high-risk central areas was an excess, not so much of low status individuals, as of persons living alone.

While these ecological studies were proceeding, other workers mounted more direct assaults on the problem of schizophrenia and social class. The existence of a steep class gradient, as gauged by first admissions to mental hospital, was confirmed in a number of countries (40, 65, 351). The most important contributions, however, came from two studies—one American, one British—which set out to relate the ecological findings to a dynamic intergeneration process.

Hollingshead and Redlich, in their survey of New Haven, Connecticut (204), carried out a survey of all cases under psychiatric treatment, together with a five percent population census of the area. They found a concentration of schizophrenia in the low social status groups, whose members were *not* more geographically mobile than others: indeed, the proportion of Class V patients who had been life-long residents in the community was higher than that of Class I and II patients. Moreover, most of the Class I and II patients had lived in the better residential quarters, and most of the Class V patients in the poorer quarters, throughout their lives; no evidence was found of a drift to the poor areas antedating the onset of schizophrenia. When the patients' social class distribution was compared with that of their parents, it appeared that over 90 percent of patients were in the same class as their families of orientation; hence, downward social mobility could hardly explain the observed gradient.

In view of the great care and thoroughness of the New Haven study, its findings were accorded a good deal of weight. Yet within a few years a strikingly different set of findings was reported by two British workers. Goldberg and Morrison compared the social class distribution for a random sample of young male schizophrenic patients with that for their fathers at the same age (149). For this purpose, they were able to use the records of the General Register Office to draw a national sample, and to classify the father's occupation at the time of each patient's birth. The results, summarized in Table XXVII, showed that although the distribution of the patients manifested the typical schizophrenic skew, that of their fathers at the same stage of life was representative of the general population.

TABLE XXVII

SOCIAL CLASS DISTRIBUTION OF SCHIZOPHRENIC PATIENTS
AND THEIR FATHERS

(Male first admissions aged 25-34 years, England and Wales, 1956)

Social Class	Patients at Admission		Fathers at Patients' Birth	
	Observed	Expected	Observed	Expected
I	12	12	14	8
II	21	44	42	42
III	178	203	192	192
IV	52	55	66	68
V	90	39	55	59
Total	353	353	369	369
Not stated	18		2	

Source: Goldberg and Morrison (149).

In a related study, the same investigators examined a series of schizophrenic patients aged 15 to 30 admitted to London mental hospitals. The patients' homes were visited to explore the socio-economic status of parents, uncles, grandparents and siblings. The findings confirmed that there had been a decline from father to son and that the patients themselves had either fallen in occupational level before hospital admission, or had never achieved the level which might have been predicted from their school careers. The social class distribution of male relatives, on the other hand, did not differ from that of the general population.

Goldberg and Morrison attempted to explain the discrepancy between their findings and those of the New Haven survey on the basis that different criteria had been used to establish social class: they had employed an index solely of occupational status, whereas Hollingshead and Redlich (204) had constructed one which also incorporated school grades and district of residence. Since non-hospitalized schizophrenics often live with their parents, the latter measure would tend to obscure intergeneration differences in occupational status. More recent American work has served to confirm the findings of Goldberg and Morrison (101), so that the present weight of evidence favours the "drift" or "segregation" hypothesis as the chief explanation of the ecological picture in schizophrenia. Although the argument is not finally settled, it seems unlikely that either social class or district of residence plays any important part in the aetiology of this disorder.

These findings in no way invalidate the research cited in Chapter 4, which has demonstrated the influence of social factors on the course and outcome of the disease. It has been shown repeatedly that schizophrenic patients of low socio-economic status are at a disadvantage as regards early diagnosis and treatment, more often become chronic hospital inmates, and fare less well after discharge from hospital than those from higher social strata (40, 73, 204). Moreover, the social class differential in outcome can be reduced by active rehabilitation policies (476).

The moral for research workers is clear: observations made on the distribution of established disease at a given point in time must be interpreted with great caution. In particular, any associations between clinical and social variables revealed in this way may or may not prove to be of causal significance. For more convincing evidence of a causal link, one must turn to longitudinal studies which can explore the association over a period of time, or even from one generation to the next. This point must also be borne in mind when studying the relationship between mental disorder and physical illness.

PSYCHIATRIC AND PHYSICAL ILLNESS

A positive association between some forms of organic pathology and of psychopathology is a basic underlying premise of psy-

chosomatic theory. The corollary of an association between manifest psychological and somatic symptoms is not necessarily implied;
some writers, indeed, have implied that the association may be
negative, since the two broad categories of symptom represent
alternative ways of reacting to stress-situations. Nevertheless, a
number of empirical studies over the past two decades have suggested that psychiatric and physical morbidity do show a tendency
to cluster together within populations. In the Baltimore survey of
chronic illness (98), a higher than average prevalence of both
acute and chronic physical disease was found among neurotic patients and their families. A survey of 1,000 American university
students found that those who had attended psychiatric clinics had
higher than average rates for various types of physical illness
(397). A number of workers have shown that clustering of all
kinds of sickness tends to occur within family groups, and that
mental illness in one member can be related to an increased incidence of morbidity in the rest of the group (50, 229, 408, 423).
Hinkle and Wolff, on the evidence of a series of studies of illness-
experience among various population subgroups, enunciated a
general theory of "illness-proneness" in the following terms:

> Those persons exhibiting the greater susceptibility to illness exhibit
> a greater susceptibility to all forms of illness, such that the greater the
> number of episodes of illness which they experience, the greater the
> number of organ systems which are likely to be involved. Those having
> the greater number of bodily illnesses are likely to experience more
> accidents and disturbances of mood, thought and behaviour (202).

Most studies in this field can be faulted for having measured
the use of medical services, rather than total morbidity. Thus, of
all persons in a community who in a given period suffer from
upper respiratory infections, those who consult on this account
will probably include an unrepresentatively high proportion of
anxious, hypochondriacal individuals. A study confined to con-
sulting patients would then suggest a link between upper respiratory infection and morbid anxiety which could well be an artefact
of the research design.

A second, related point is that in many studies which seek to
test associations between physical and psychological disorders,

both are expressions of a single latent variable, namely the patient's own perception of his state of health. A great deal of medical diagnosis depends heavily upon the patient's reporting of symptoms; in minor ill-health, especially, there may be little in the way of confirmatory physical signs or laboratory findings. Since depressed or anxious patients tend to complain of a variety of somatic symptoms, and to perceive themselves as unhealthy, they have a greater than average probability of being given organic diagnoses. Here again, the effect on any enquiry that depends on symptom-reporting will be to create a spurious association between physical and psychiatric illness.

The first of these difficulties can be overcome by using indices of morbidity which are independent of medical consultation. The Baltimore survey of chronic sickness, for example, was based on regular home visiting of a random sample of the local population (98) . Some investigators have made use of health diaries in which members of population samples are asked to keep a complete record of all ill-health and medical complaints for an agreed period of time. This approach has the advantage that untreated episodes can be identified, and the individual's contacts with medical services related to his background of minor ill-health. Moreover, an adult subject can be asked to record the illness-episodes of other members of his family, so that the total family experience of morbidity can be examined.

Brown (41) , using this technique, compared the illness-experience of a sample of neurotic married women and their families with that of a matched control group of families drawn from the same general practice population. The findings are summarized in Table XXVIII.

The neurotic patients and the controls were found to differ in respect of self-reported morbidity, as well as in frequency of medical consultation; a weighted "illness-score" based on the severity and duration of symptoms showed a highly significant difference between the two groups. Differences between the husbands were less pronounced, but here again the index group reported a higher number of days unwell. Finally, the index-group children had more consultations, more days unwell and more re-

TABLE XXVIII
COMPARISONS OF FAMILY ILLNESS-EXPERIENCE OF NEUROTIC
MARRIED WOMEN AND OF MATCHED CONTROLS DURING ONE YEAR

Index of Morbidity	Neurotic Group	Control Group	Probability Level
Patients:	(n = 32)	(n = 32)	
Mean number of medical consultations	8.7	3.1	0.01
Mean number of illness-episodes	5.3	3.9	0.01
Mean number of days with medical symptoms	106	60	0.01
Husbands:	(n = 32)	(n = 32)	
Number diagnosed as neurotic	15	2	0.01
Mean number of days with medical symptoms	95	58	0.01
Children:	(n = 55)	(n = 56)	
Mean number of medical consultations:			
Boys	4.4	3.8	N.S.
Girls	4.6	2.5	0.05
Mean number of days with medical symptoms:			
Boys	72	49	0.05
Girls	81	51	0.01

Source: adapted from Shepherd *et al.* (423).

ported neurotic traits than their controls. That all these differences showed up more strongly among the girls presumably relates to the fact that the groups had been defined in terms of the mothers' mental health: studies based on other sampling criteria have indicated that boys are at least as vulnerable as girls to pathogenic influences in the family (409).

Findings of this kind strongly suggest that the apparent clustering of physical and mental illness within populations cannot be explained solely in terms of differential use of medical services. They do not, however, meet the objection that the patient's self-perception may still be an important source of bias. To settle the point, investigators will have to use morbidity indices based on objective data; in particular, on observations which are independent of the patients' reporting of symptoms. This is not an easy condition to meet, but some progress has been made by a recent health survey in southeastern England (103) .

As part of a research programme in preventive medicine, a screening project was set up in a community health centre. The survey sample comprised all patients between forty and sixty-five years in a large group practice; but as the survey formed part of a controlled evaluative study, only half the patients, randomly selected, were invited to attend for check-up. Eventually, 1,500 patients, or 70 per cent of those eligible, took part, a proportion which, although it compares favourably with many prescriptive screening programmes, indicates the limitations of this method of case-detection.

The screening procedure comprised three stages. First, each patient underwent a battery of physical and chemical tests, including visual testing, audiometry, blood-pressure reading, body-fat measurement, spirometry, electrocardiography, urinalysis, and various blood tests. Second, at a separate appointment a week or two later, each patient was examined physically by his family doctor and his health reviewed in the light both of this examination and of the test results. Third, wherever the possibility of undiagnosed disease was raised either by the test findings or by physical examination, further investigations were made.

A multiphasic screening process of this type can serve to detect unsuspected disease, and to assess the individual's state of health independently of his complaints or contacts with medical services. It thus has great value for the investigation of psychophysical relationships, provided an independent psychological assessment can be made. In the present instance, each patient completed a questionnaire containing 20 items from the CMI Health Questionnaire known to discriminate between neurotic and normal subjects (104) . All those with five or more positive responses were regarded as probable psychiatric cases, and examined by a psychiatrist using a standardised interview procedure (148) . For each confirmed case, a matched control was then drawn from among the patients who had no positive questionnaire responses; each provisional control patient likewise underwent a standard psychiatric interview.

By this method, it was possible to match two contrasting groups of patients: one with definite evidence of psychiatric morbidity, the other free from psychiatric symptoms or disability. The two groups were inspected for any differences in physical health as shown by the results of the screening programme. For this purpose, the survey findings for the two groups were organized in a number of ways; for example, as the mean values of various physiological indices; as the mean number of individual diagnoses; and as the relative frequency of major, minor and psychosomatic illness. Somewhat unexpectedly, the largest intergroup differences were found in the frequency of major illness: that is, of conditions which might be expected, if unchecked, to shorten life. Minor ill-health and psychosomatic affections did not show such clear-cut differences between the two groups; nor were the mean values for blood-pressure, vital capacity and other physiological variables significantly different. Table XXIX summarizes the findings for cardiovascular disease, where the greatest disparities were found.

TABLE XXIX

DISTRIBUTION OF MAJOR CARDIO-VASCULAR DISEASES AMONG
MIDDLE-AGED PSYCHIATRIC PATIENTS AND MATCHED CONTROLS

Cardiovascular Disease	Males		Females	
	Index	Control	Index	Control
	%	%	%	%
None	62.0	86.5	69.0	84.0
Coronary artery disease	27.1	10.8	18.5	9.2
Hypertension	5.5	2.7	6.9	3.4
Hypertension and coronary artery disease	2.7	—	3.5	2.3
Congenital/rheumatic heart disease	—	—	1.1	1.1
Peripheral vascular disease	2.7	—	—	—
Total	100.0	100.0	100.0	100.0
No. of patients	37	37	87	87

Source: Eastwood (103).

This study suggests that the association between physical ill-health and psychiatric disorder cannot be explained wholly in terms of the self-perceptions of neurotic patients. Nor does it appear to be restricted to those conditions commonly described as "psychosomatic"; rather it seems that the whole spectrum of chronic major illness may be involved.

Once again, the need for cautious interpretation must be stressed. One has to bear in mind that 30 percent of the population at risk failed to attend for screening, and that this group may have contributed a serious element of bias. Furthermore, since the survey findings did not distinguish between known disease and that previously unrecognized, it is not clear how many of the index and control patients had been aware beforehand of the presence of morbidity. Presumably some at least of the index group were depressed or anxious because of such awareness.

These considerations underline the case for research in which the development of physical illness can be related chronologically to changes in the mental state, and both viewed against the background of the person's social situation. We do not yet know how often and how closely psychiatric disturbance precedes major physical illness; how often it is secondary, and if the association between the two can be explained in terms of differential experience of stress-situations. Cohort studies are needed to establish how far the course and outcome of physical disease are psychologically determined. In short, the investigation of clinical, as of socio-economic, correlates of mental disorder points unequivocally to the importance of longitudinal surveys, which can examine biological and environmental factors operating both before and during illness. Statistical associations can be tested most readily for those changes which occur immediately prior to illness-onset, and hence may be regarded as precipitants thereof.

PRECIPITATING FACTORS

The progress of research on this subject has been impeded by the theoretical notions of "reactivity" held by different schools of psychiatry. European authorities have tended to reserve the term "reactive" for circumscribed groups of mental disorder which they regard as distinct clinical entities; thus, reactive, or psychogenic, psychoses are held to be separate from the main body of psychotic disorders (115); in particular, schizophreniform reactions have been distinguished from true, or "process" schizophrenia (264). In the United States, different concepts have held sway. Many psychiatrists, influenced by the teaching of Adolf Meyer, have preferred to speak of "reaction-types" rather than of disease entities; others, mostly psychoanalysts, have questioned the value of any system of formal diagnosis. British psychiatry has been influenced by both the European and the American traditions, as the long-standing dispute over the classification of depression bears witness (234).

The criteria for "reactivity" have been poorly defined and unsystematically applied. Jaspers (217) laid down that there should be a clearly adequate precipitating factor closely related in time to the onset of illness; that the psychological content of the illness should be manifestly related to this factor, and that recovery should follow on its removal. Not many psychiatric disorders fulfil all three criteria; indeed, the nearer any individual reaction approached to doing so, the less likely would it be to gain recognition as pathological.

Few systematic studies have been undertaken on the proximal causes of any form of mental illness. Evidence on reactivity has come from two principal sources: first, studies of populations or large groups exposed to acute environmental stress; secondly, controlled studies of events anteceding the onset of acute psychiatric disturbance. A third source, that of experimental studies, has contributed some indirect evidence, but is beyond the scope of this review.

Studies of Acute Stress-Situations

In modern times, the most dramatic illustrations have come from military sources. British experience in the First World War led to official recognition of the importance of psychiatric casualties for the armed forces; as a result psychiatrists played a much more prominent part in the second conflict (5). They were not slow to grasp the effect of battle conditions on the psychiatric rates:

> The numbers correlate indirectly with the surgical casualties—following about three days behind the curve of daily incidence. But it is not a parallel curve; as the surgical casualties rise, the psychiatric

losses rise out of all proportion. Dependent on the type of battle, two per cent to thirty per cent of all casualties may be psychiatric (301).

In the United States Army, careful and systematic recording likewise revealed a close relation between the psychiatric and the surgical casualty rates (141). Figure 11 illustrates the close correlation which was found between battle injury and psychiatric casualty rates occurring in three divisions of the 5th United States Army during a seven-week period of active service. The relationship remained fairly constant throughout at one psychiatric admission to every four or five troops wounded in action.

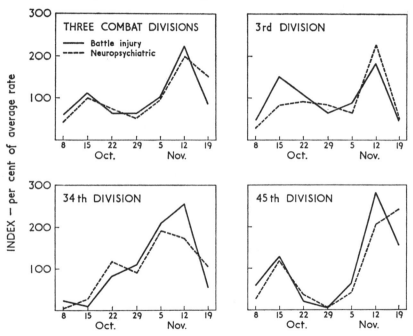

Figure 11. Relation between trend of battle injury and neuropsychiatric admissions, selected divisions, Fifth U. S. Army. Source: Glass and Bernucci (141).

Under peacetime conditions, the effects on exposed populations have been documented for a variety of forms of social change, including migration, displacement, social mobility, economic cycles and, most notably, rapid processes of acculturation

(338) . In view of the problems of method in this field of enquiry, none of these studies can be regarded as definitive.

Earlier research suggested that mental illness-rates among immigrant groups in different countries were greatly in excess of those of the indigenous populations (64, 463) . The classic investigation by Ødegaard (349) revealed a higher rate of mental hospital admission among Norwegian immigrants in Minnesota than among the native-born population; moreover, the rate was even higher among those migrants who returned to the home country. Ødegaard, like a number of other workers, explained his findings in terms of a selective tendency for vulnerable or unstable individuals to leave their own country and hence to be found disproportionately among immigrant groups. More modern studies have largely failed to confirm this pattern, until it can be said that "Today the relationship [between mental illness and emigration] has become quite doubtful, and its meaning equally so" (338) . The shift may have resulted partly from changes in immigration policy, including more careful screening of prospective immigrants. Undoubtedly, it has been due in some measure to more sophisticated research techniques; Malzberg (304) , for example, found that when the rates for immigrants in New York State were standardized for such factors as urban/rural distribution, differences from the indigenous population became negligible.

The highest rates of mental disorder have been found in those immigrant groups such as refugees and displaced persons whose migration could scarcely be classed as voluntary (109, 377) . In this context it is virtually impossible to differentiate between what Murphy (338) has described as the four interlocking factors of loss of homeland, experience of persecution, cultural difficulties of readjustment and social isolation. Even when emigration occurs under strong political pressures, as after the Hungarian uprising of 1956, there is still a selective tendency for unstable, prepsychotic individuals to join the exodus (326) .

More compelling evidence of the reactive nature of mental illness has come from research on those types of life-change with a major biological component. As a rule, such changes cannot be observed in the mass, but have to be monitored as they occur in the life-span of susceptible individuals. Two examples which serve to illustrate the general theme are child-bearing and surgical operations.

Childbirth and Mental Illness

Childbirth, by reason of its physiological, psychological and socio-cultural aspects, can be seen as the paradigm for a stress-situation. At the same time, as a readily identifiable point-event, it lends itself to epidemiological enquiry. It is, therefore, remarkable how few population studies have been undertaken on this subject.

In one such investigation (383), data on mental hospital first admissions in Massachusetts during 1950 were related to estimates of the general population of women aged fifteen to forty-five years, according to defined childbearing status in that year. Comparison of the observed and expected numbers of first admissions revealed a large increase for psychosis, and a smaller increase for nonpsychotic disorders, during the three months postpartum. Admission rates for both these categories remained high over the ensuing six months, although significantly so only for the psychotic group. The findings are summarized in Table XXX.

Comparable findings were reported from a survey of Hamilton County, Ohio (357), which reviewed the obstetric records of all women aged fifteen to forty-five years who were patients in any of its psychiatric hospitals between 1940 and 1958. Events of pregnancy, labour and the puerperium were also compiled for women of the same ethnic status, delivered in the same maternity unit immediately before and after each psychiatric patient. Comparison with this normal control group showed that postpartum psychosis was associated with a number of obstetric and perinatal complications, and also with a history of previous psychiatric illness; hence, both precipitating and predisposing factors were implicated. The results thus bore out the conclusion by Seager (419), on the basis of his own controlled study, that the puerperium is a stress-situation which can trigger off various forms of mental illness in susceptible women. Figure 12 clearly demonstrates the temporal relationship of parturition to the onset of mental illness.

TABLE XXX

OBSERVED AND EXPECTED NUMBERS* OF FIRST ADMISSIONS TO MENTAL HOSPITALS AMONG THE MARRIED CHILDBEARING POPULATION (MASSACHUSETTS, 1950), ACCORDING TO STAGE OF CHILDBEARING AND CATEGORY OF PSYCHIATRIC DIAGNOSIS

Stage of Child-bearing	Month	Number Observed	Number Expected	Chi-Square Value†	p Value
Psychoses:					
Pregnancy	0-2	1	6.3	2.89	0.10-0.05
	3-5	1	6.3	2.89	0.10-0.05
	6-8	—	6.3	4.42	0.65-0.02
After delivery	0-2	30	6.4	85.99	0.001
	3-5	10	6.4	1.55	0.30-0.20
	6-8	10	6.4	1.55	0.30-0.20
Other diagnoses:					
Pregnancy	0-2	2	4.1	0.49	0.50-0.30
	3-5	—	4.1	2.90	0.10-0.05
	6-8	1	4.1	1.44	0.30-0.20
After delivery	0-2	9	4.2	4.43	0.05-0.02
	3-5	6	4.2	0.41	0.70-0.50
	6-8	6	4.2	0.41	0.70-0.50

*Observed and expected in 40 percent of admissions
†All values for chi square based on Yates correction for small expected numbers
Source: Pugh *et al.* (383).

Postoperative Reactions

Major surgery is another biological event whose effects upon the mental state form a potentially rewarding subject for research. Here again, the number of population-based studies has been small, perhaps because of the difficulty of estimating rates for a defined population (247). Disease classifications do not list postoperative psychosis as a separate entity; since the clinical picture is variable, cases are assigned to a number of diagnostic categories and the official returns cannot be used to calculate prevalence rates. Moreover, few general hospitals serve clearly-defined base-populations; in cities, for example, the pressure on beds often results in patients being admitted to units at some distance from their homes. Finally, because the less severe cases are unlikely to be transferred to psychiatric care, their enumeration will depend on the recognition of mental disturbance by surgeons and nurses, and upon the willingness of these workers to cooperate in any enquiry.

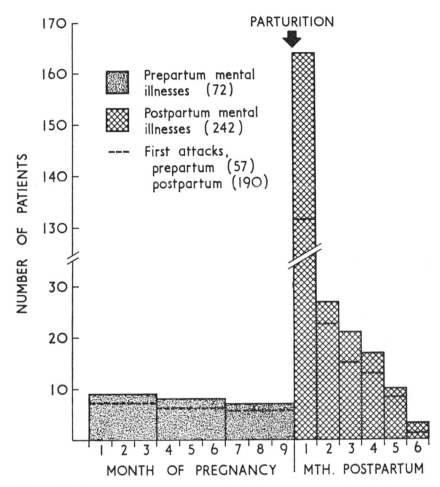

Figure 12. Onset of parapartum mental illnesses among hospitalized patients in Hamilton County, Ohio, 1940-58. Source: Paffenbarger (357).

In a survey of Belfast hospitals, Knox (247) overcame some of the more serious problems of method. All psychiatric referrals could be traced; the parent population was geographically stable, the distances involved small, and the surgical statistics reliable. The rate for postoperative psychiatric illness severe enough to lead to specialist referral was one in 1,600, the clinical picture ranging from acute confusional states to schizophrenia and affective psychosis. The findings were in broad agreement with those of earlier surveys which had reported an average rate for postoperative psychosis of about one in 1,500 cases (274) .

Hysterectomy has long been reputed to have a high incidence of psychiatric sequelae. The literature on this subject is not easy to interpret: case-criteria have ranged from mental hospital admission to mild emotional instability; the case-series have tended to be small, and inception rates have seldom been calculated for defined populations. It is not surprising, therefore, that the reported findings have varied between a very low rate of complications (189) and an incidence amounting to 30 percent of all cases (3). The retrospective survey by Barker (17) , using data from the Dundee Case-Register, represents an advance on previous studies. All psychiatric referrals were entered on a central record, so that case-enumeration was simple and age-specific referral rates could be calculated for the base-population. A total of over 700 hysterectomies performed in four years was abstracted from local hospital files, and the psychiatric register searched for evidence of referral of any of the women concerned during a follow-up ranging from two to seven years. The control group was made up of women from the same population who had undergone cholecystectomy during the survey period. Psychiatric referral was found to have been three times as frequent among the posthysterectomy group as among the controls, whose rate was average for the population.

Barker's study emphasizes the importance of an extended follow-up period, a point whose neglect may explain some of the inconsistencies in earlier findings. It remains true that studies which employ psychiatric referral as the case-criterion will detect only the more severe postoperative disturbances. In order to provide a balanced perspective, it will be necessary to undertake prospective studies in the community, with routine follow-up of all cases.

Studies of Antecedent Events

In clinical psychiatry, the traditional approach to the question of reactivity has been through the individual biography, or "life-chart" (324) , in which major life-events are plotted against the occurrence of illness episodes. This method can serve as a useful epidemiological tool where adequate records are available: a situation which may obtain in industry (202), in the armed services (384) and—potentially, at least—in general practice (229). The consensus of findings from these sources has been that illnesses are not randomly distributed over the life-span, but occur in clusters of up to two or three years' duration. Such clusters can be related to periods of environmental change and individual difficulties of adaptation. Holmes and his co-workers have attempted to quantify life-change according to prevailing cultural standards, and have reported a positive correlation between annual morbidity-experience and the corresponding total of "Life Change Units" (384).

A more precise technique for studying the relationship between environmental change and the acute onset of mental illness has been developed by two British workers (42). By means of a careful check of all events and changes which had occurred over a three-month period, they were able to compare the recent life-experience of a sample of patients admitted to hospital for acute schizophrenia with that of a large group of normal controls. The findings, illustrated in Figure 13, showed that the index group had experienced a sharp increase in the number of life-events, including those of a fortuitous nature, during the three weeks prior to the onset of acute symptoms.

Although research of this kind deliberately focuses on the immediate precursors of illness, it may incidentally point to the equal importance of predisposition. Indeed, no aetiological model in psychiatry can be regarded as complete unless it pays attention both to proximal and to distal causative factors.

PREDISPOSING FACTORS

The primary influences bearing on the individual's expectancy of mental disorder are to be found in his genetic endowment, the nature of his biological environment in utero and during infancy, and the socio-cultural factors which determine his early learning experiences. Epidemiological surveys have contributed to knowledge in each of these areas, of which the genetic is undoubtedly the best charted.

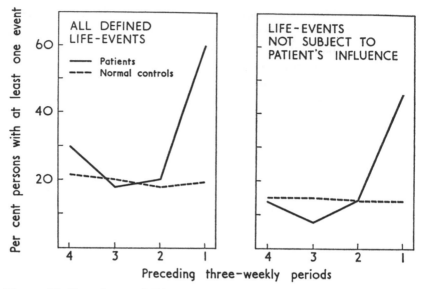

Figure 13. Experience of life-events during four consecutive three-weekly periods. (a) 50 patients immediately prior to onset of schizophrenic illness. (b) 325 Normal controls immediately prior to interview. Source: Derived from Brown and Birley (42).

Genetic Studies

The earliest workers sought to ascertain the amount of "hereditary tainting" in the general population. In so doing, they paid little attention to the need for sampling techniques, accurate diagnosis, and stratification by age and degree of consanguinity (447). Strenuous efforts to overcome these defects were made by Rüdin and his followers of the Munich school, who tried to elucidate genetic patterns of morbidity by relating concordance rates among the relatives of psychotic patients to the degree of consanguinity, and to expectancy rates in the general population (426). The concept of the empirical genetic prognosis (empirische Erbprognose) was introduced, whereby a number of propositi were chosen as randomly as possible and the incidence of various traits ascertained among first-degree relatives, and in some instances among collaterals: the resulting incidence rates were then compared with those for the relatives of abnormal propositi. The need was recognized to distinguish clinical forms of psychiatric abnormality, and to eschew the ill-defined notion of "tainting" used in earlier studies. These workers also introduced the concept of "expectancy," or risk of developing a given disease during the individual's lifetime.

Inevitably, most studies of consanguinity had to be based on relatively small samples, of the order of 100 to 200 propositi. Nevertheless, the overall rates obtained by combining these samples have provided useful estimates of morbid expectancy, as can be seen from Table XXXI.

TABLE XXXI

FREQUENCY OF SCHIZOPHRENIA IN THE GENERAL POPULATION AND IN THE RELATIVES OF SCHIZOPHRENICS: POOLED DATA

No. of Investi- gations	No. of Coun- tries	Relationship to Schizophrenic	No. of Relatives Investigated (Corrected)	Expectation of Schizophrenia in %
19	6	Unrelated (gen. popn.)	330,752	0.86
14	8	Parents	6,622	5.07
12	7	Sibs.	8,484.5	8.53
6	2	Children	1,226.5	12.31
4	4	Uncles and aunts	3,376	2.01
5	4	Nephews and nieces	2,315	2.24
4	4	First cousins	2,438.5	2.91
		Twin Pairs:	Both twins affected	
6	5	DZ (opp. sex)	24/430	5.6
9	7	DZ (same sex)	71/593	12.0
10	8	MZ	252/437	57.7

Source: Shields and Slater (427).

More accurate expectancy rates might be anticipated from cohort studies. Klemperer (244), a pioneer of this technique in psychiatry, set out to trace 1,000 persons born in Munich between 1880 and 1890, but succeeded in locating only 70 percent of the total. Fremming (128) achieved a better result by studying the more static population of the Danish island of Bornholm; here he was able to trace over 90 percent of all persons born in the period

1883-1887. The expectancy rates of 0.9 percent for schizophrenia and 1.6 percent for manic-depressive psychosis, which he estimated, must be seen in relation to the size of the island population (5,500 all told) and its presumably unrepresentative gene-pool. Nevertheless, a large cohort study in Iceland, undertaken along similar lines, yielded broadly comparable findings (191).

The assessment of genetic factors in mental illness has come to be seen as a highly complex issue. To regard the occurrence of morbidity in families as a direct expression of biological inheritance is now recognized as a gross oversimplification. Wender and his co-workers have put the point aptly:

> Interpretation of increased incidence [of schizophrenia] in families is difficult because the deviant psychological experiences have usually been received at the hands of the patient's biological relatives. It is impossible to decide the extent to which the disturbance in schizophrenic offspring has been genetically or psychologically determined, since the deviance in the parents' child-rearing techniques may be the manifestation or forme fruste of schizophrenic illness in the parents, rather than the cause of illness in the child (464).

Twin studies, long regarded as the key to this problem, have tended to lose favour in recent years. Psychodynamic theory has emphasized the complex psychological forces peculiar to the twin situation; to the extent that these forces pose each twin a special problem of identity, they may be thought of as exercising an influence on the risk of schizophrenic illness (213). The too-sweeping claims of earlier population geneticists, and the notable discrepancies in more recently reported concordance rates, have alike provided ammunition for hostile critics. The earlier population studies, which reported strikingly high monozygotic concordance rates (221, 289) have been heavily criticized for inconsistency of case-definition and inadequate sampling methods. Rosenthal (401), in the course of a detailed critique, has suggested that the importance of genetic factors may be exaggerated by hospital-based studies, and that future research should focus on representative population samples.

Two recent Scandinavian studies paying regard to this precept have reported low schizophrenic concordance in twins. Kringlen

(255), using the Norwegian birth-register and National Register of Psychosis, examined all twin-pairs between thirty-five and sixty-five years, one or both of whom had a history of functional mental illness: the age-range was chosen on the assumption that most of the sample would have passed through the peak risk-period for schizophrenia. Detailed zygosity rates were calculated, using blood groups in 70 percent of cases. The monozygotic concordance was estimated at 28 to 38 percent, and the dizygotic at 5 to 14 percent. Kringlen's findings led him to conclude that the more careful and accurate the sampling technique, the lower the reported concordance. An even more striking result was obtained by Tienaari (453), who in a study of over 2,000 twin pairs born in Finland between 1924 and 1929 found none concordant for schizophrenia. Tienaari discarded half of his sample on the grounds that one or both of the twins had died, a procedure not without danger of bias, insofar as mental disorder and institutional care may be associated with early death. His findings in consequence must be viewed with some caution, though they certainly cannot be dismissed.

More recent attempts to disentangle genetic and environmental influences have made use of the process of adoption. Heston (195) carried out a controlled study of a group of adults who had been born to schizophrenic mothers and permanently separated from them within two weeks of birth. In this way, he planned to test the genetic contribution to schizophrenia independent of any effects of upbringing by a psychotic parent. His experimental group comprised all persons born to schizophrenic mothers between 1915 and 1945 in Oregon State Psychiatric Hospital, where separation from the mother soon after birth was mandatory. The findings showed a significant excess of schizophrenic and sociopathic disorders in this group when compared with matched controls also reared in foster-homes.

A series of studies initiated by the National Institute of Mental Health, Bethesda, has provided strong confirmatory evidence that schizophrenia has a genetic basis. The Adoptive Parents Study (464) employed a questionnaire survey of psychiatrists in the eastern states of the United States to identify adults, aged fifteen to thirty-five years, who had been adopted in the first year of life,

TABLE XXXII
PSYCHIATRIC DISORDERS IN FOSTER-HOME REARED SUBJECTS

Psychiatric Disorder	Propositi (Schizophrenic mothers)	Controls (Normal parents)	Exact Probability
Schizophrenia	5	0	0.024
Mental subnormality	4	0	0.052
Sociopathic personality	9	2	0.017
Neurotic personality disorder	13	7	0.052
No. of cases	47	50	
Mean age at follow-up	35.8	36.3	

Source: Heston (195).

had at some time been diagnosed as schizophrenic, and had shown no evidence of organic cerebral disease. As judged by psychological test results, combined with clinical assessment, the biological parents of this group showed significantly more psychiatric disturbance than did the adoptive parents. Making allowance for any bias inherent in the method of case-collection, it is hard to gainsay this finding. In the Extended Family Study (241), thirty-seven persons diagnosed as schizophrenic were identified from the list of over 5,000 adoptions recorded in the Copenhagen Adoption Register between 1924 and 1947. This group was compared with a matched control group of adoptees who had no history of mental hospital admission. A large excess of schizophrenic illness was found in the biological families of the index group, as against the families both of their adoptive parents and of the control group. Here again, the findings are difficult to explain on any basis other than the genetic transmission of some factor predisposing to schizophrenia.

In summary, most of the evidence continues to point to the importance of hereditary factors in schizophrenia, and to a lesser extent in other forms of major mental illness; nevertheless, the effect of introducing epidemiological principles into this field of research has been to reduce the genetic component to size, and by so doing to redirect attention to the part played by the environment.

Prenatal and Paranatal Factors

If the role of hereditary transmission has still to be clearly defined, that of prenatal and paranatal influences remains largely a mystery. The relation of central nervous damage in the child to maternal infections, metabolic disorders and immunological reactions is well established (295). On the other hand, there is little agreement about the implication of such factors in functional psychiatric disorder.

The pathogenic significance of prenatal and paranatal factors was investigated by Pasamanick and his co-workers on the following hypotheses:

> Inasmuch as prematurity and complications of pregnancy are associated with foetal and neonatal death, usually on the basis of injury to the brain, there must remain a fraction so injured who do not die; depending upon the degree and location of trauma they go on to develop a series of disorders extending from cerebral palsy, epilepsy and mental deficiency through all types of behavioural and learning disabilities which are a result of lesser degrees of damage sufficient to disorganize behavioural development and lower thresholds to stress; and further, these abnormalities of pregnancy are associated with certain life-experiences, usually socio-economically determined, with the consequence that they themselves and their resulting neuro-psychiatric disorders find greater aggregation in the lower strata of our society (360).

This theory postulates a "continuum of reproductive insult" and a corresponding spectrum of reproductive casualty ranging from death, through varying degrees of neuropsychiatric disorder to minor behavioural disturbance. Seven different clinical entities have been studied; namely, epilepsy (281), cerebral palsy (282), tics (362), speech disorders (361), reading disabilities (224), behavioural disorders (363) and mental deficiency (245). Of these, only the last two will be discussed here.

In their initial, retrospective, study of mental deficiency, the investigators reviewed hospital obstetric records, noting any association of deficiency with premature birth, maternal complications of pregnancy, neonatal abnormalities, socio-economic status, race and season of birth. They then proceeded to an anterospective study, in which five hundred premature infants were compared with a control group of full-term infants, matched for hospital of birth as well as for socio-economic circumstances (245, 246). At forty weeks, the premature infants showed a higher incidence of neurological abnormality, and a lower average quotient on the Gesell Development Examination; moreover, the degree of abnormality was proportional to that of prematurity as judged by birth weight.

The differences were confirmed when three hundred of the children were re-examined two years later; but by this time there was evidence of divergence between the white and coloured children, who at forty weeks had been equal in performance. Whereas the white children now showed an improvement in adaptive and language skills, the opposite was true of the coloured children, the most marked decline having occurred in those whose mothers had poor educational records. This divergence was attributed to the differing socio-cultural expectations of the two ethnic groups.

The distribution of premature births and complications of pregnancy for the survey sample as a whole showed a preponderance in the lower social status groups, a finding, summarized in Table XXXIII, which led the investigators to suggest that obstetric complications should be considered as possible aetiological factors whenever the incidence of neuropsychiatric disorder differed markedly between ethnic and socio-economic groups.

TABLE XXXIII

INCIDENCE OF PREMATURITY AND COMPLICATIONS OF PREGNANCY, BY SOCIAL CLASS AND ETHNIC STATUS

Socio-economic status	Prematurity	Paranatal factor Bleeding Toxaemia	All Complications
	%	%	%
Highest group	5	5	5
Lowest group*:			
White	7.6	14.6	10
Non-white	11.4	50.6	15

*10 percentile groups for prematurity; 20 percentile groups for bleeding and toxaemia, and for all complications combined.
Source: Knobloch and Pasamanick (245).

Behavioural disorders were examined by a retrospective study of children referred to the Special Services Division of the Baltimore Department of Education (363, 398). Controls, selected from the school class-lists, consisted in each instance of the next child in alphabetical order, of the same sex and ethnic status, born in Baltimore. The city birth-registers were combed for information about parents, socioeconomic status and place of birth. For those born in hospital, obstetric data were obtained, including any history of complications of pregnancy or delivery, birthweight and neonatal progress. The behavioural disorder cases were found to have three times the incidence of prematurity for the controls, and an excess of complications of pregnancy ranging from 125 to 150 percent. On the other hand, they had no higher rates of difficult, prolonged labour or of operative procedures at delivery; nor was any difference found between index and control groups with regard to family composition and the age, education, employment and housing conditions of the parents.

These latter findings, being based on a hospital-based, retrospective enquiry, must be considered tentative. Nevertheless, the highly significant differences which were found suggest the probability of a real association between childhood behavioural disturbance and a history of obstetric complications. The underlying mechanisms are not clear, although Pasamanick's suggestion of undiagnosed minimal brain damage has to be taken seriously.

In the long term, anterospective studies will be required to elucidate the problem. One British study, based on a stratified sample of children born during one week in 1946 (406), has already added to our knowledge of the neuropsychiatric sequelae of prematurity. The original sample contained just over 700 infants with birth-weights of $5\frac{1}{2}$ lb. or less; in the ensuing years, this group was examined periodically for any developmental abnormalities. Douglas, who conducted the enquiry, believed that major deficiencies of method in earlier studies threw doubt on their conclusion that children born prematurely suffered no handicap unless they showed clear evidence of brain damage (97).

All the premature infants for whom socio-economic data were available were matched by age, ordinal position, maternal age, social class and home conditions with full-term infants drawn from the same sample. When these matched pairs were compared at eight years on a battery of psychometric tests, the index children gained lower average scores than the controls. A second assessment at eleven years, combined with educational reports and teachers' ratings, showed the premature children still at a serious disadvantage (96). By this time, however, their handicaps were at least partly attributable to poor home circumstances; for, despite the initial matching, many differences had developed between the index and control groups: differences which became more pronounced as the study went on. Douglas' own assessment agreed with those of teachers and public health nurses in suggesting a relative lack of concern for their children's welfare among the index-group mothers. Furthermore, the index-group fathers had had more spells of unemployment than their counterparts, and showed a relative decline in socio-economic status.

Broadly similar findings were reported by Drillien (99, 100), who studied a cohort of premature children in Edinburgh. At two years, the most premature group (birth-weight $4\frac{1}{2}$ lb. or less) contained a striking excess of developmentally retarded children, as judged by the Gesell Development Examination. Drillien also reserved judgment on the relative importance of premature birth and the poor maternal care and home conditions with which it tended to be associated.

There is thus an outstanding need for further prospective studies of this subject, in which variables such as socio-economic status can be adequately controlled. Meanwhile, prevalence survey findings have provided some support for Pasamanick's hypothesis of a continuum of reproductive casualty. A survey of schoolchildren in the Isle of Wight (412) identified neurological and psychiatric disorder independently, and revealed a strong positive association between the two.

Even though severely handicapped children had been automatically excluded from the sample, it appears that children with some evidence of brain damage contributed disproportionately to the total psychiatric prevalence. In particular, their psychiatric rate was three times that for children with other kinds of physical handicap: a highly significant difference.

TABLE XXXIV

PREVALENCE OF PSYCHIATRIC DISORDER IN NEURO-EPILEPTIC
CHILDREN AGED 5-14 YEARS ATTENDING SCHOOL

	With Psychiatric Disorder		Total
	No.	*%*	
General population (10- and 11-year-old children)	144	6.6	2,189
Physical disorders not involving brain	16	11.5	139
Blind only	1	16.6	6
Deaf only	2	15.4	13
Lesion at or below brain stem	2	13.3	15
Miscellaneous other physical disorders*	11	10.3	107
Brain disorder	34	34.3	99
Uncomplicated epilepsy	18	28.6	63
Lesion above brain stem (but no fits)	9	37.5	24
Lesion above brain stem (with fits)	7	58.3	12

*This group includes 2 children who also have lesions below the brain stem
Source: Rutter, Graham and Yule (412).

Some at least of the psychiatric disorder among the neuro-epileptic children thus appeared to be a direct consequence of cerebral dysfunction, rather than of the psycho-social stresses entailed by any form of chronic ill-health or handicap. Although no prevalence survey can establish causal relationships, the findings in this instance were consistent with Pasamanick's viewpoint.

Environmental Factors in Early Life

The role of early parental loss as a pathogenic factor has received much prominence over the past twenty years, partly as a result of Bowlby's work. In his WHO monograph (34), he emphasized the child's need for "a warm, intimate and continuous relationship with his mother, or permanent mother substitute, in which both find satisfaction and enjoyment," opining that the lack of such a relationship could have an ominous significance for future mental health.

This hypothesis in its original form has been subjected to a good deal of critical scrutiny; notably by Wootton (482), whose opinions on this—as, indeed, on other psychiatric topics—command respect as those of an exceptionally shrewd, well-informed lay person. Most research on parental deprivation, as she was quick to point out, has been seriously deficient both in criteria and in methodology. Deprivation cannot be treated as a unitary concept, because the significance for the child will depend upon its age at the time, the cause of loss or separation, the nature of the parent-child relationship, and the extent to which other adults can fill the breach. Psychological rejection has to be distinguished from physical separation, with which it by no means always coincides. Separation and loss due to unavoidable circumstances may have consequences very different from desertion, cruelty or neglect.

Emotional disturbance is all too common among children in hospitals and institutions; but as the effects of parental deprivation cannot be disentangled from those due to the institutional regime, it is no surprise that conflicting findings have been reported. Thus, Bowlby's early work was not confirmed by Hilda Lewis, who followed up 500 children for two to three years after their admission to a reception centre. Nearly one-third of the children removed from their mothers made a satisfactory adjustment; nor was a worse outcome noted for those separated before the age of two. Lewis concluded that:

> . . . unduly dogmatic statements about the ill-effects of maternal deprivation often leave out of account the emotional hazards and harms children may suffer from bad mothers and indifferent mother-substitutes, or the variety of sources (including the father) from whom children may draw love and support necessary for their happiness (279).

The difficulties involved in population-based research on this topic are formidable. Bowlby himself, comparing epidemiological and clinical strategies, commented some years ago that his own research group had abandoned the former but found the latter much more rewarding. The comparison is misleading, since these different approaches are complementary not alternative: studies of the effects of separation on the individual child, though essential, cannot answer basic questions about the aetiological significance of this experience. The distributions in the general population of both psychiatric disorder and early parental loss must be known before any association between the two can be established.

Despite the difficulties, substantial progress is now being made in this direction. A body of evidence has accrued in recent years which links early parental loss to the risk of mental illness in adult life. The findings for schizophrenia have been equivocal, but it seems unlikely that parental deprivation will prove an important predisposing cause of this condition (197, 354). Stronger indications have been found of an association with depressive illness (92, 200), while parental loss during childhood has also been shown to increase the risk of later suicide (47, 167).

In view of the many intervening variables which must be controlled, few if any of the published studies can be taken as definitive. Apart from the usual problems of demographic matching, investigators have to take account of ordinal position and of parental age at the time of birth (164). The expectancy of orphanhood varies over the years and from place to place (169, 92), so that reliance on national vital statistics may be misleading. Most studies have been retrospective, and few have employed truly representative samples. Even where an association is demonstrated, it may not be causal: the incidence of suicide, for example, is much higher than average in the families of manic-depressive patients (443, 374); in this instance, early parental loss may be associated with suicidal behaviour as the result of a genetic predisposition.

There is a pressing need for anterospective studies which will allow childhood experience to be monitored systematically. The handful of such enquiries so far undertaken have already yielded valuable information on the natural history of childhood disorders, and to a lesser extent on the relationship of childhood experience to adult disorders (395). Thus, the Berkeley Growth Study assessed a random sample of Californian children at yearly intervals from birth up to the age of fourteen (293). The British National Survey of Child Health followed up a cohort of children born during one week in 1946. After four years, no significant difference in emotional disturbance was found between those children who had lost one parent and a matched control group with no such experience of loss (405). A later controlled study of the same sample (97) showed only small increases among the index group of such symptoms as nightmares and thumb-sucking.

A number of cohort studies have shown associations between delinquency and the quality of the early home environment (143, 315): findings which have been explained in terms of the psychology of character development (368). On this basis, some workers have constructed predictive scales of delinquency which can be applied during the early years of childhood (144). Although such instruments carry a grave danger of misapplication, they may be of service in directing attention to the need for social measures.

In England, the Cambridge Study in Delinquent Development (466) has confirmed by a prospective enquiry that bad home circumstances in early life greatly increase the risk of future delinquency. The sample comprised all eight-year-old boys attending six primary schools in a working-class area of London. After six years, searches at the Criminal Records Office and at local children's departments established that of the total of 411 boys, thirty (7.3%) were early delinquents. A further eighty-seven (21.2%) were classed as unofficial early delinquents on the evidence of reports from teachers, neighbours or parents. Table XXXV summarizes the association between home conditions, assessed at the start of the survey, and subsequent delinquency.

An alternative strategy which can sometimes be employed is the systematic study of groups who are known to have undergone standardized psychological testing. An outstanding instance was a study of former university students known to have committed suicide (358), in which the investigators had access to routine test data. At the University of Pennsylvania, the college case-records over the ten year period 1931-1940 gave the responses of all students to a questionnaire enquiry on nervous symptoms and personality traits. The responses of fifty students who later com-

TABLE XXXV
EARLY DELINQUENCY IN RELATION TO SOCIAL HANDICAP

Items of Social Handicap	Status of Boy on Records of Early Delinquency							
	Convicted Delinquents (N = 30)		Reported Delinquents (N = 87)		Non-Delinquents (N = 294)		X² value	P <
	n	%	n	%	n	%		
Supported family	16	53.3	33	37.9	34	11.6	51.1	0.001
Low occupational status of father	9	30.0	12	13.8	44	15.0	4.97	0.10
Poor housing*	18	66.7	35	40.7	81	27.7	19.8	0.001
Poorly kept accommodation*	10	37.1	10	12.2	30	10.3	16.1	0.001
Inadequate income*	18	66.7	29	34.5	43	15.1	45.2	0.001
Six or more children	15	50.0	15	17.2	37	12.2	36.0	0.001
Boy physically neglected*	12	42.9	14	16.7	23	8.0	25.7	0.001

The percentages show the proportion of boys in each of the categories of early delinquency who were subject to the item of handicap indicated.
*On these variables a few (< 16) of the 411 boys were not rated.
The percentages and chi-square comparisons refer to the known cases only.
Source: Gibson and West (140).

mitted suicide were compared with those of one hundred controls, two students from the same intake being randomly selected to match each index case. The results are given in Table XXXVI.

Information of this kind falls into the predictive category already discussed in relation to individual prognosis and morbid risk. In addition, it is directly relevant to questions of aetiology. When the sample was augmented by a comparable group of former Harvard students, the index and control subjects were found to be alike in respect of family social status, number of siblings and size of community of residence, and to have come equally from urban and rural backgrounds. They differed, however, in some important familial characteristics: significantly more often, the index-group students at entry to university had reported separation of the parents, death of the father or ill-health of the father. Death or ill-health of the mother did not appear to distinguish between the two groups. Here, in short, the combination of opportunity and careful research design established the role of certain family influences as risk-factors for suicide, while at the

TABLE XXXVI
COMPARISON OF QUESTIONNAIRE RESPONSES OF STUDENTS WHO
LATER COMMITTED SUICIDE WITH THOSE OF A RANDOM CONTROL
GROUP (UNIVERSITY OF PENNSYLVANIA, 1931-40)

Item	Percentage of Affirmative Responses		P
	Suicides (N = 50)	Controls (N = 100)	
Instruction: Place a tick mark after those conditions to which you are subject and a 0 after those which you never have			
Sensation of heart beating	20	14	0.34
Nervousness	28	17	0.12
Insomnia (sleeplessness)	16	6	<0.05
Sense of exhaustion	16	12	0.49
Instruction: Put tick after affirmative Replies, 0 for negative			
Are you subject to worries?	50	29	0.01
Are you particularly self-conscious?	42	20	<0.01
Are you bothered by a feeling that people are watching or talking about you?	20	8	0.03
Are you subject to moods?	40	30	0.21
Are you subject to periods of alternating gloom and cheerfulness?	46	31	0.07
Are you inclined to be secretive and seclusive?	22	10	<0.05
"Anxiety-depression index"*	30	10	<0.01

*Affirmative responses to five or more of the above items
Source: Paffenbarger and Asnes (358).

same time yielding a glimpse of the underlying psychological mechanisms.

This chapter has given some indication of the wide range of epidemiological research which has already contributed to our knowledge of the causes of mental disorder. While substantial progress has been made, it is clear that the epidemiological approach has been limited both by a lack of integration with other research strategies and by its own serious methodological deficiencies. Further achievements will depend increasingly upon the development and application of scientific survey techniques; it is, therefore, to a consideration of the outstanding problems of method that we now turn.

Chapter Six

THE IMPACT OF MODERN TECHNIQUES

INSPECTION OF THE METHODS and scope of epidemiological psychiatry has highlighted two major obstacles to further advance. First, there is a continuing lack of objectivity in case-identification which leaves investigators, in the words of Lewis, "hampered and sometimes nonplussed by the fact that diagnostic procedure and the details of clinical examination are not safely comparable" (275). Secondly, the epidemiological approach is still relatively isolated from other research strategies in psychiatry. Future progress will depend largely upon the success with which this isolation can be overcome. Epidemiology, as Terris has remarked,

> must utilize both observational and experimental studies . . . it needs to operate . . . in close collaboration with clinical and laboratory personnel and facilities. Finally, it should not hesitate to use all scientific methods, whether derived from the natural or the social sciences, which can be helpful in determining and explaining the behaviour of specific diseases in the population (449).

Of recent years, workers in this field have become increasingly conscious of the needs for a more rigorous scientific methodology. Such attempts as have been made to forecast the development of the subject have served chiefly to emphasize the same point. The most pressing need today remains that defined by a WHO Expert Committee in 1960:

> . . . the development of technical methods and concepts applicable either in the preliminary studies which yield hypotheses or in the more closely defined studies which attempt to put these hypotheses to the test (483).

Research into methods and concepts subsumes a wide range of studies concerned with the standardisation of clinical measures, the application of psychological, biological and socio-cultural indices, and the use of modern techniques for data analysis. The present chapter can provide no more than a brief review of some of the more important developments in these fields.

137

ADVANCES IN CLINICAL DEFINITION

Over the past decade, much attention has been devoted to the construction of standard classifications of mental disorder. The subject is of direct relevance for the epidemiologist, whose chief concern is to find a system acceptable to his clinical colleagues which is at the same time appropriate for survey research.

If agreement is to be reached on terminology, operational definitions are essential. A notable advance has been made by the publication of disease glossaries, which are intended to reduce ambiguity and to facilitate communication (441). The psychiatric glossaries in official use in the United States (9) and in Great Britain (137) bear witness to the amount of agreement possible, even among psychiatrists of widely differing background and orientation. Nevertheless, the two manuals reveal some important differences of outlook. The British, based on the 8th Revision of the *International Classification of Diseases* (484), deliberately avoids broad definitions of psychosis and neurosis. The American manual, bolder in this respect, serves to illustrate the difficulties of the subject. While its formulation of psychosis is purely descriptive, that given for neurosis invokes causal mechanisms:

> Anxiety is the chief characteristic of the neuroses. It may be felt and expressed directly, or it may be controlled unconsciously and automatically by conversion, displacement and various other psychological mechanisms. Generally, these mechanisms produce symptoms experienced as subjective distress from which the patient requires relief (9).

It has already been argued in Chapter 2 that a definition couched in such terms is of limited value for empirical research. To function effectively, a glossary must rely as little as possible on theoretical doctrines, however compelling. There are some indications that the point has now been taken, and that future editions of both glossaries will concentrate increasingly on the phenomenology of disease.

The two manuals also differ in their commentaries on the major psychiatric syndromes. Thus, the American definition of schizophrenia employs terms of low operational utility, such as alteration of concept formation, psychologically self-protective delusions and loss of empathy; whereas the British definition places the emphasis on such universally recognized features of the disease as auditory hallucinations, ideas of influence and thought disorder. That these are not merely academic issues is shown by the very large differences between the two countries' reported rates for schizophrenia and affective psychosis (80).

Research workers have reported a number of difficulties in using each of these glossaries. Wing, for example, has described some of the problems which arise in the analysis of case-register data (478). In the *International Classification of Diseases,* Involutional Melancholia still appears as a separate entity, distinct from Manic-Depressive Psychosis (depressed type); yet the glossary descriptions of these two conditions are for practical purposes indistinguishable. Some categories are based on phenomenology; others on causal factors. When two members of the committee which compiled the British glossary were asked to categorize a patient whose schizophreniform illness had been precipitated by heavy drinking, one suggested the label of Schizophrenia, the other of Alcoholic Psychosis.

Many psychiatric patients cannot be adequately classified under a single diagnostic label. Wing (478) reported that one-quarter of her case-register sample were best defined by using two diagnostic terms. The system which she has developed for statistical purposes permits up to three psychiatric syndromes to be recorded on computer-tape, according to a hierarchy of clinical importance and severity. Any known or suspected causal factor is also coded and placed on the same tape; a separate code is given for mental subnormality, whether or not related to the psychiatric disorder. Finally, any additional physical abnormality not directly related to the psychiatric condition can also be coded and given a special position on the computer-tape. The following case-examples illustrate the use of the method.

1. An illness with symptoms characteristic of schizophrenia (paranoid type), clearly precipitated by greater than usual alcoholic excess in a man who was a habitual heavy drinker, and who had an aggressive personality.

Classification

Underlying or precipitating cause	Alcohol
1st psychiatric condition	Paranoid schizophrenia
2nd psychiatric condition	Habitual excessive drinking
3rd psychiatric condition	Aggressive personality
Mental subnormality	—
Additional physical illness or handicap	—

2. A child who was severely subnormal because of phenylke-tonuria, with a psychotic behaviour disorder *not* autistic or schizophrenic in nature.

Classification

Underlying or precipitating cause	Phenylketonuria
1st psychiatric condition	Childhood psychosis, other
2nd psychiatric condition	—
3rd psychiatric condition	—
Mental subnormality	Severely subnormal
Additional physical illness or handicap	—

This multiaxial system permits clinical phenomena and causal factors to be recorded independently, in a manner which would be impossible with the traditional form of classification. The tri-axial system for coding childhood psychiatric disorders, recom-mended by a WHO study group (413), relies on similar princi-ples, although in this instance "underlying cause" and "addition-al physical conditions" are combined under a single code.

Diagnoses, being abstractions, tend to be recorded less reli-ably, even with the aid of a standard classification, than the in-dividual symptoms and behavioural abnormalities from which they are derived. A recent international diagnostic exercise (421) showed a high degree of concordance in the rating of psychiatric symptoms, despite much diagnostic disagreement. Hence, symp-tom and behaviour rating-scales may convey more reliable information than diagnostic labels: a point of some importance for case-enumeration.

A standardized psychiatric interview which incorporates symptom-ratings cannot automatically provide the appropriate diagnosis for each patient. It can, however, help to narrow the range of disagreement among clinical psychiatrists; it can also be adapted for purposes of numerical taxonomy (435). Standardized interviews thus have distinct advantages for group research, provided they match the requirements of survey technique.

The construction of such an instrument demands careful analysis of the normal diagnostic process. Spitzer and his co-workers, in developing their "Psychiatric Status Schedule" (437, 438), laid down a set of precepts in relation to the consecutive stages of clinical assessment, as follows:

1. *Deciding what has to be measured.* Only that information should be considered which is directly relevant to diagnosis, prognosis or the assessment of severity, and which can be both clearly defined and reliably recorded. At this stage, possible aetiological factors should be ignored.

2. *Obtaining information and eliciting behaviour.* Interview techniques are to be preferred as a means of obtaining the necessary information, because they combine flexibility with maximum coverage, while at the same time permitting the continuity and rapport of a good clinical examination.

3. *Making the judgment.* At this stage the risk of error due to observer-bias must be considered. Such error can be reduced with the aid of an initial period of training for the interviewers, in which joint-interviews and videotape techniques are used. Any consistent bias thus revealed can be obviated, or at least corrected statistically.

4. *Recording the judgment,* and

5. *Summarizing the findings quantitatively.* The data obtained at interview should be recorded and scored on pre-coded sheets which include specific item-scales. Additional comments by the interviewer will often prove valuable if the score-sheet is to serve as a clinical record.

This approach has been developed most comprehensively by Wing and his colleagues, whose "Present State Examination" (473) calls for an essentially clinical technique. The interview concentrates on symptoms experienced during the preceding month, any earlier psychiatric history being the subject of separate enquiry. The use of mandatory questions enables those areas which require more detailed probing to be outlined; the interviewer is then free to ask as many questions as he wishes to establish whether or not any given item should be rated positively. In this respect, the method represents an important departure from that of Spitzer's group, in which there is no free probing and each response has to be taken at face value. Despite its high degree of flexibility, the Present State Examination has proved reliable under test conditions (235, 474). It has not been used in epidemiological studies and for this purpose will require modification, having been designed primarily for use with hospital patients.

A standardized psychiatric interview designed specially for community surveys has been described by another British group (148). The principal requirements for its construction were held to be as follows:

1. The assessment should be made by an experienced psychiatrist in a realistic clinical setting;
2. The interview should be acceptable to people who do not regard themselves as mentally or emotionally disturbed;
3. The interview's content should be appropriate for the types of psychiatric disorder commonly encountered in the general population;
4. The interview should generate information about individual symptoms and signs of morbidity, as well as an overall diagnostic assessment;
5. It should discriminate clearly both between mentally disturbed and normal individuals, and between patients with different degrees of mental abnormality;
6. It should be economical of time, so as to allow large numbers of persons to be interviewed;

7. The psychiatric assessment and clinical item ratings should be reliable in the sense of being reproducible by different trained observers.

The interview schedule, which is used in conjunction with a detailed instruction manual, allows the examiner freedom to probe as necessary to elicit the duration, frequency and severity of symptoms or morbid states. It has a number of possible applications apart from case-identification; for example, it has been employed to test for associations between clinical and social variables in controlled studies (76, 103), and as a means of rating change in psychiatric state over time (147).

Although clinical interview procedures are relevant mainly to the second stage of case-identification, the two terms cannot be equated. Nonclinical techniques of measurement, such as Guttman scaling of symptoms (212), may play a part at the second stage, if only as adjuncts to clinical assessment. Conversely, first-stage screening tests are frequently based on clinical criteria.

Some screening techniques consist of observation and recording by physicians, or by ancillary staff under their supervision. In other instances, non-medical personnel act as key informants, whose information is sifted and evaluated by medical investigators. In some situations, and for certain types of disorder, this represents the most effective—possibly the only—method of case-identification. A case in point, already cited, is the reporting of heroin-users by fellow addicts under treatment (6); other relevant examples include the recognition of disturbance in school-children by their class teachers (142, 411, 425) and of alcoholism in the employed population by industrial management (188). Any such screening procedure must satisfy ethical requirements as well as meeting the standards of validity, reliability and specificity already outlined.

PSYCHOMETRIC TESTS OF ILLNESS AND DEVIANCE

In modern industrial society, psychiatric screening is frequently based on some form of standardized psychometric test. It is convenient to distinguish between clinical and psychometric methods, although the difference is one of emphasis rather than of substance. The term clinical has been used here to refer exclusively to methods based on the examination of individuals, or the evaluation of case-material, by medically-trained investigators. The term psychometric will be used for those techniques based on the administration of standardized tests, or on self-administered tests, which do not rely on the making of clinical judgments. This dichotomy ignores the potential role of the clinical psychologist in epidemiological research, a role which has still to be defined (79).

A distinction must also be drawn between those tests which detect or measure *illness* and those which purport to delineate *personality*. While the former are more obviously relevant to the problems of epidemiology, the latter, as we shall see, do have a part to play in this field of research.

Most of the earlier tests made use of imperfectly calibrated scales based on self-administered questionnaires. The Cornell Medical Index (CMI) Health Questionnaire has been widely employed as a measure of psychiatric disturbance (39, 85), although it was not originally intended for this purpose and in practice has serious defects. Its low sensitivity is revealed by the finding of one study that 30 percent of a psychiatric out-patient sample scored below the recommended cut-off point (423). In the same investigation, patients' scores were found to be inversely related to their socio-economic status; while a high test-retest correlation after one year suggested that responses were being heavily influenced by personality traits, as distinct from illness.

More recently, a number of attempts have been made to construct symptom inventories free from such blemishes. The Middlesex Hospital Questionnaire (83) consists of a 48-item self-rating scale which yields a symptom profile along six subscales (free-floating anxiety, phobic, obsessional, depressive, hysterical and somatic symptoms). Originally designed for hospital studies, this instrument has now been shown to discriminate between neurotic patients and a putatively normal group (84), so that it may prove useful for community surveys. Another recently developed inventory, the Symptom Rating Test of Kellner and

Sheffield (230), was designed primarily to measure clinical change in response to treatment, but has proved effective in discriminating between psychiatric out-patients, neurotics under general practitioner care, and healthy normals.

Goldberg's General Health Questionnaire (146) is noteworthy for the care with which it has been designed and validated. Intended to pick out non-psychotic psychiatric illness, it is applicable in clinical work, community surveys or longitudinal studies aimed at assessing clinical change. By permitting a graduated response to each item, it avoids the errors inherent in bimodal response scales, while at the same time allowing any given response to be classed as normal or morbid. The wording of the items places the emphasis throughout on current ill-health rather than on personality factors.

Starting with 140 items culled from a number of symptom inventories, Goldberg used three calibration groups: One hundred non-psychotic patients in mental hospital wards ("severely ill"); one hundred psychiatric out-patients ("mildly ill") and one hundred persons selected from the general population by a stratified sampling technique, and confirmed as being in good health ("normal"). Once all poorly discriminating items had been discarded, the instrument was found to have high test-retest and "split-half" reliability. Validity was assessed for samples of medical out-patients and general practice patients, by correlating the questionnaire scores with independent clinical ratings. In these sub-studies, less than nine percent of the respondents were misclassified by the questionnaire. Re-administration after some months showed that patients' scores varied in keeping with changes in their clinical condition, suggesting that the results were not seriously affected by personality factors. On all these counts, the General Health Questionnaire represents a distinct advance over most of the earlier screening tests.

Personality measures, such as Cattell's 16 PF Questionnaire (60, 61) and the Eysenck Personality Inventory (114), are akin to complaint-inventories in being simple pencil-and-paper tests which can be administered to large numbers and hence are practicable as screening instruments. To the epidemiologist, however, they are useful only as subsidiary tools which may help to relate the known distribution of morbidity in a given population to sub-clinical variants and personality deviance (177, 184). So far, it must be said, this approach has yielded slender returns.

Paradoxically, the use of personality measures has proved more rewarding in studies of physical morbidity, where it can provide a valuable tool for psychosomatic research. Such studies, having a firm anchor in organic pathology, escape the excessive dependence on verbal techniques of those which endeavor to relate personality to psychiatric illness.

In recent years, a good deal of attention has been focussed on the role of personality and behavioural factors in the aetiology of heart disease. Conflict in the reported findings can be ascribed largely to defects of research method (300). In this field, prospective studies have been much the most convincing; hence the great interest aroused by the work of the Western Collaborative Group (400). In a prospective study of some 3,500 subjects, 70 developed clinical or electrocardiographic evidence of coronary artery disease during a two-year risk period. The most important predictive factor appeared to be a well-defined behaviour pattern ("Type A"), associated with driving, ambitious character traits and a highly-developed sense of time and urgency. The presence of hypertension and of lipoprotein abnormalities in the blood were predictive of ischaemic heart disease only insofar as these factors were associated with Type A behaviour.

These findings have been criticized as unreliable, the behavioural typology not being based on standardized psychological tests. More recent work, however, suggests that Type A behaviour can be reliably identified (219). Moreover, other anterospective studies have supported the view that personality traits are linked with the risk of coronary disease. One such investigation (433) followed up two samples of students: a high-risk group with raised serum cholesterol and positive family histories, and a low-risk group with abnormally low serum cholesterol levels. According to the 16 PF Questionnaire (60), members of the high-risk group were aggressive, anxious and self-critical; while those in the low-risk group tended to be easy-going, friendly and self-satisfied. In another study (356), nearly 2,000 men were followed up for four years, after an initial assessment based on the Minnesota Multiphasic Personality Inventory (187) and the 16 PF Questionnaire (60). Those who developed angina pectoris had shown the most deviant scores on the HS and Hy scales of the MMPI and on the C scale of the 16 PF Questionnaire. These findings were considered to show that the risk of angina was positively related to emotional lability and a low tolerance for environmental stress.

Not all research findings on this topic have pointed in the same direction. In one study designed to test the behavioural hypothesis, the incidence of behaviour-type A among patients with coronary artery disease did not differ significantly from that in a healthy control group (227). Another enquiry (211) distinguished four groups by clinical diagnosis, or degree of risk based on blood pressure and serum cholesterol values. Only patients with established coronary disease showed the expected combination of high anxiety and depression with low hostility scores on the MMPI. Patients in the "high-risk" group actually showed a reversal of this pattern in their personality profiles. The conclusion was reached that personality deviance as assessed by such methods is more likely to follow than to precede the onset of ischaemic heart disease.

Studies of this kind underline the importance of distinguishing primary psychological factors from those secondary to physical disease: hence the need for long-term prospective studies of random population samples. The investigations cited above show a welcome movement in this direction, although some problems of method remain to be solved. Apart from the standardization of personality and behavioural measures, variables such as diet, exercise, genetic and endocrine factors must be considered if consistent results are to be achieved. In short, this area of research exemplifies the general trend in psychiatry towards the correlation of standardized psychological and biological indices.

THE USE OF BIOLOGICAL INDICES

Hitherto, cytological, biochemical and physiological tests have been used in psychiatry mainly to confirm clinical diagnosis, rather than as screening instruments. Increasingly, however, as new, rapid and economic laboratory techniques become available, such tests are likely to play their part in screening programmes. Although it is too early to say which will find wide application, a number are already gaining in prominence.

Cytogenetic Studies

Chromosomal abnormalities have assumed importance in the study of mental retardation, developmental sexual anomalies and antisocial behaviour. One group of workers (81) has shown that it is feasible to apply cytogenetic techniques in population surveys; for example, the technique of blood culture, whereby lymphocytes are stimulated to synthesize DNA and then to divide, is easily standardized and can be successfully carried out on a general practice population (82). The need is well recognized to obtain chromosome pictures from representative samples, both to determine the total prevalence of constitutional abnormality and to assess the proportion of abnormal karyotypes in phenotypically normal individuals. To judge from one survey in which 20,000 infants in maternity units were examined by means of buccal smear techniques (294), it appears that 2.1 per 1,000 male live-births are associated with some type of sex chromosome abnormality. Institutional studies suggest that those affected may be at increased risk both for mental retardation and for behavioural disorders.

Cytogenic studies of delinquent groups seem destined to increase our understanding of some aspects of antisocial behaviour. There is no doubt that men with XXY, XY/XXY, XXYY and XYY sex-chromosome complements are present in greater than expected numbers in institutions for mentally disordered offenders. Some evidence suggests that whilst XXY complement affects intelligence primarily, the XYY complement may be associated with antisocial behaviour even in the absence of intellectual defect (58, 346).

Although a good deal is now known about the chromosomal aberrations in Down's syndrome (mongolism), there remains a need for studies of their distribution in the general population, and of the extent to which the familes of those affected show cyto-genetic or other abnormalities (67). The clinical observation of a link between Down's syndrome and leukaemia (256) has led to population-based surveys of leukaemia among the parents of mongol children (203) and among mongols in different environ-ments (214).

Geneticists are keenly aware of the enormous scope for research opened up by the cytological advances of the past twenty years (373), and some disappointment has been evinced that so few psychiatrists have shown active interest in a subject which may have profound implications for their work (122).

Biochemical and Chemical Techniques

Biochemical tests have found little place in psychiatric screen-ing; partly because of the technical difficulties; partly because of the dearth of established biochemical correlates of mental dis-order. So far, their main sphere of application has been in the study of mental retardation. A large number of inborn metabolic errors are now known to be associated with mental defects: they comprise amino-acid disorders such as phenylketonuria and ho-mocystinuria; lipid disorders such as gargoylism and Tay-Sachs disease; and carbohydrate disorders such as galactosaemia and fructosaemia (461). For the most part, these conditions are too rare to justify prescriptive screening programmes. In some in-stances, however, simple, rapidly administered tests are available, the most notable example being the detection of phenylketonuria in newborn infants. In Great Britain, routine testing by public health nurses of some 850,000 infants identified 39 previously un-suspected cases (322). Whatever the efficacy of dietary measures, this approach to presymptomatic diagnosis is potentially of the greatest significance for prevention.

Biochemical studies of functional mental illness have so far paid disappointingly small dividends, in part because of the pit-falls of method to which all cross-disciplinary research is subject. Few clinical psychiatrists can hope to assess critically the pro-cedures employed by their colleagues in the laboratory; converse-ly, biochemists quickly find themselves lost in the complexities of psychiatric diagnosis. Neither group may be expert in survey methodology. Under the circumstances, it is perhaps not surprising that confusion should have arisen.

The controversy over the "pink spot" in schizophrenia epitomises this kind of difficulty. In the early 1960s, a number of conflicting reports appeared (130, 376). One series of experiments (32) purported to show that the "pink spot" on urinary chromatography was typical of patients with "first-rank" symptoms of schizophrenia, and seldom found in conjunction with other forms of mental disorder, or among normal people. In these investigations, however, the index group had been drawn from the patient-populations of three mental hospitals, many being chronic inmates; the principal control groups, in contrast, were made up of healthy individuals (mainly university staff and students) and patients in general hospital beds. Environmental factors such as diet could not, therefore, be adequately controlled. Subsequently, other workers reported that the pink spot was to be found in only a minority of schizophrenic cases, and was actually more frequent in Parkinson's disease (262). It now seems probable that this phenomenon is related to dietary factors, rather than to the biochemistry of schizophrenia (375).

If biochemical tests are usually inappropriate for surveys of the general population, some have a special role in the screening of high-risk groups. Institutional populations, for example, are subject to nutritional deficiencies which in turn may have adverse effects on the mental state. It has been remarked that mental disorders are now more likely to be associated with vitamin B_{12} deficiency than with a positive serological reaction for syphilis; hence an easily applied screening test, comparable to the Wassermann reaction, is required (261). Since, however, low vitamin B_{12} and serum folate concentration can occur in the absence of anaemia, peripheral blood films may be inadequate for screening purposes. Biological assay techniques, on the other hand, are well standardized and can provide sensitive indices of the underlying pathology.

A Norwegian survey (108) found that of all patients admitted to a mental hospital during one year, 5.8 percent had vitamin B_{12} concentrations below the critical level for pernicious anaemia. British surveys (193, 209) have reported a much lower incidence of B_{12} deficiency; on the other hand, low serum folate levels were found in no less than 35 percent of patients admitted to a psychiatric unit (209). Surveys of psychogeriatric populations have revealed an even higher incidence of vitamin deficiency (428).

An association is now well established between low serum folate levels and long-term medication with barbiturates and anticonvulsant drugs. Epileptic patients thus constitute another high-risk group for folate deficiency, and for related mental changes which are potentially reversible (392). The anti-folate effect of alcohol (194) renders chronic alcoholics liable to the same changes.

The development of rapid, reliable screening procedures is crucial for research on those high-risk groups which come under surveillance only briefly and at critical periods. The need for sensitive chemical tests of alcohol in the body is well-recognized in relation to traffic accidents. It has been estimated that a raised blood alcohol concentration is present in either the driver or the victim in about half the 50,000 fatal traffic accidents which occur annually in the United States (158). The use of a breathalyser test in a controlled study of road accidents in Grand Rapids showed clearly that the risk of casualties rose sharply above a blood alcohol concentration of 0.04 gm percent (30). Further research is urgently needed into many aspects of this major social problem.

The current issue of narcotic addiction among United States service veterans returning from Vietnam also raises political and social questions of great consequence. The difficulties of screening large numbers of veterans is obvious, particularly where failure to distinguish chemically between addictive drugs and other ingested substances could result in a high proportion of "false positives": nevertheless, the public health implications are too serious for the problem to be ignored. With the development of automated test procedures, the screening of large contingents is now becoming a practical proposition.

Urinary adrenal steroid excretion has been examined in persons subjected to psychological stress, such as ambulance men during wartime combat (33) and parents of children with neoplastic disease (131). Little or no relation was found between the degree of stress and the level of steroid excretion, and it was concluded that man is capable, at least temporarily, of making a good physiological adaptation to most stress-situations. The lowest levels of steroid excretion occurred in those persons who made the most pronounced use of psychological defence mechanisms; for example, parents who denied to themselves the gravity of their children's illnesses.

Measures of steroid excretion are at best a general index of arousal, and cannot be regarded as screeening tests for specific psychiatric syndromes. They may find some application in screening certain types of risk-group, such as men in the armed services, with a view to predicting responses under acute stress conditions. In this context, however, direct physiological measures afford greater promise.

Physiological Measures

Measures of physiological disturbance are potentially among the more reliable screening procedures. Doubts about their role in epidemiological research stem partly from questions of practicability; partly from the imperfect correlation of physiological and psychological variables. There are inherent dangers in what has been termed the "substitution game" (321) of using chemical or physiological indices, which are relatively easy to standardize, instead of clinical observations, which are not so. Just as the serum cholesterol level cannot be taken as a gauge of ischaemic heart disease, so no physiological variable directly reflects psychiatric morbidity.

From this point of view, the most valid procedures yet available are those in which measures of physiological arousal are used to monitor changes in the level of fear and anxiety. Simple measures such as the pulse rate and blood pressure lend themselves most readily to the epidemiological approach. More sophisticated techniques usually have the drawback of being too cumbersome and time-consuming for large-scale field studies. Measurement of forearm blood flow, for example, has proved effective in hospital studies (231), but would be difficult to adapt for population surveys. Electrical skin conductance, which provides another useful correlate of anxiety (259), is more promising in that it can be registered by an easily transportable polygraph: it has been used, for instance, to study arousal in men making parachute drops (118). Nevertheless, this technique also presents difficulties of method and interpretation which must be overcome before it can be employed as a screening instrument.

The same considerations apply *a fortiori* to the use of the EEG in population surveys. Besides being an expensive and laborious technique, electro-encephalography is essentially an adjunct to clinical assessment. Thus, a survey of the elderly population of a mental hospital (460) concluded that although EEG readings could differentiate between normal cerebral function and gross organic deterioration, they were of no value in distinguishing mild or borderline cases. The efficiency of this procedure as a test for dementia was poor, recordings being at times normal in cases of obvious dementia, and at other times abnormal in patients with no serious impairment.

In the absence of major technological advances, the EEG seems destined for use as a screening instrument only in certain clearly defined situations involving known high-risk groups. One such situation arises in genetic research: the EEG has been utilized to detect cerebral dysrhythmia in the relatives of epileptic patients since the pioneer work of the 1930s (272, 445). Metrakos (323) found an EEG reading suggestive of centrencephalic epilepsy to be a much stronger hereditary trait than the occurrence of epileptic seizures; he postulated a dominant autosomal gene with penetrance determined by age, rising from almost zero at birth to a maximum between four and sixteen years, and then declining. There is ample scope for research in this field, particularly in familial studies of EEG abnormality and psychiatric disorder.

A second context of some importance for psychiatry is the detection and monitoring of cerebral dysfunction following head-injury (89). Routine electroencephalography may find useful application in studies of "post-traumatic neurosis" and of the morbid risk for post-traumatic epilepsy and other long-term sequelae. It can also be of service in the periodic examination of boxers who are at risk for traumatic encephalopathy (267).

Finally, the EEG retains a position in research into aggressive criminal behaviour. A number of electro-encephalographic studies of murderers (199, 416, 480) have reported a preponderance of abnormal readings among those found insane, or whose crimes were apparently motiveless; on the other hand, those with clear motivation showed no higher rates of abnormality than the general prison population. In a recent study of a large sample of violent criminals, Williams (469) found abnormal EEG patterns in 65 percent of habitual offenders, compared with only 24 percent who had committed single acts of violence. On present evidence, therefore, EEG abnormalities are associated both with impulsive homicide and with repeated aggressive behaviour. In studies of non-violent offenders and juvenile delinquents, electro-encephalography has proved of little or no discriminatory value (468).

MEASUREMENT OF ENVIRONMENTAL FACTORS

Any population group is exposed not only to a range of noxious and pathogenic agents, but also to certain conditions of geophysical habitat, climate and natural resources which will serve to determine its total mortality and morbidity experience during a given period. Equally important is the socio-cultural environment, since in psychiatry, as Galdston has remarked, ". . . . . the physician intercedes between, not only man and nature, but most often and mainly, between man and society" (133).

The environmental factors of modern life form a constantly changing pattern, slow-moving as a rule, but at times abrupt and dramatic. Provided these factors can be identified and their strength measured, it becomes possible to examine relationships between changing conditions and the incidence of mental disorder. There are strong grounds for monitoring the effects of any sudden events, natural or man-made, which disrupt the life of a community and cause repercussions on human health and behaviour. With this point in mind, a WHO Expert Committee advocated:

> the development of frames of reference, theory and hypothesis so that more efficient use can be made of naturally occurring events . . . . By posting observers at strategic points, a research team could take advantage of a fleeting opportunity according to a pre-arranged plan (483.)

Although the importance of such opportunities for the epidemiologist can hardly be overstated, it has to be recognized that the situation following a disaster may be anything but favourable for research. Of the Peruvian earthquake in 1970, it has been commented that:

> . . . the problem was simple: to bring immediate succour to the injured, the homeless and the hungry—but how many, where and how? . . . almost every proposed solution was arguable on medical, logistic or humanitarian grounds, using arguments often, if not usually, based on faulty information (390).

Decisions regarding the procurement of supplies, setting up of field hospitals, provision of shelter for the homeless, and prevention of infectious disease assume crucial importance immediately after a disaster; in such circumstances there may be little or no place for the research worker.

Once the acute situation has been resolved and the provision of basic services is adequate, research into the sequelae of disaster becomes feasible. The 1968 floods in Bristol, England, provided an opportunity for a controlled study, since the flooded areas of the city could be clearly demarcated and matched with comparable unaffected areas. Bennet, comparing persons from flooded homes with a control group (25), found that the former experienced significantly more morbidity during the ensuing twelve months. Attendances at general practitioners' surgeries rose by 53 percent; hospital referrals and admissions more than doubled. Furthermore, mortality rates compiled for all the flooded areas of Bristol showed a 50 percent increase over the same period: a rise not reflected in other parts of the city.

Recently, similar investigations have been undertaken into the effects of social upheaval on mental health. Civil disturbance and rioting is an increasingly common feature of modern urban life, and one whose impact on psychiatry requires to be examined. Some evidence has been adduced that the Belfast riots of 1969 were followed by an increase of psychiatric morbidity, principally acute situational reactions (126, 290).

It may be predicted without undue pessimism that the scope for such enquiries will be enlarged, not merely by the increasing prevalence of civil unrest, but by new forms of communal disaster in the wake of technological advance: crashes involving giant airliners and high-speed trains; explosions in fuel depots and high-pressure gas-mains; the collapse of multi-storey buildings; the escape of radio-active and toxic substances. Moreover, less dramatic changes in man's natural and social environment are being constantly wrought by technology. There is some indication, for example, that the growing problem of aircraft noise is affecting mental health: a higher-than-expected rate of mental hospital admission has been reported from one area near London Airport subjected to intermittent high noise levels (1). Nor is the significance of rapid socio-cultural change confined to its possibly pathogenic effects; in some instances such change might equally well be predicted to lead to a decrease in psychiatric morbidity.

The monitoring of socio-cultural change is only one aspect of the wider problem of measuring the influence of social factors. The criteria, concepts and definitions entailed by sociological research are not less complex than those of psychological medicine. Moreover, current theories and types of analysis in the social sciences have not as a rule been developed with an eye to the problems of epidemiology. There is a pressing need for research on the classification and measurement of all social factors which may bear on morbidity in the general population.

The significance for mental health of the mass media of communication has attracted a wealth of speculation but surprisingly little scientific enquiry. Television is now a major socio-cultural influence on child development, comparable in importance with the neighbourhood and the school, and far outweighing the church. A number of surveys in the United States have revealed that children of school age spend an average of not less than twenty hours weekly watching a "staple fare of plays—chiefly Westerns, crime and adventure" (201). The impact of this new force on child health and behaviour calls for intensive study. The effect of newspaper reporting on imitative behaviour has been repeatedly questioned throughout this century, especially with regard to suicide. Recently, Motto (336) has reported that a prolonged newspaper "blackout" in one large American city was accompanied by a marked temporary fall in the local suicide rate; the fall was greatest among young women, the most suggestible group of the adult population. These and other instances support the case for controlled anterospective studies of possible relationships between mental health and mass communication.

Such findings also suggest a need for matching research into the communication of deviant behaviour through personal contact. Variations in psychiatric prevalence among ethnic and socioeconomic groups may reflect the communication of cultural attitudes and behaviour patterns. In large cities, immediate neighbourhood ties have been partly replaced by "social networks" (31), which are often geographically extensive. To meet this situation, the social orbit of an index group can be operationally defined in terms of first-degree relatives and close friends (381). The findings will be meaningful only if they can be related to those for matched control groups or, failing that, to reliable statistics for the parent population. The latter method is exemplified by a recent study in Edinburgh, which ascertained the incidence of suicidal attempts among the immediate relatives and friends of a sample of attempted suicide patients admitted to hospital (254). The observed frequency was significantly in excess of the expected figure, based on the known demographic and ecological pattern of attempted suicide for the city. Whatever hypotheses are put forward to explain this association, the empirical finding opens up a promising new line of enquiry.

The social network, the extended family and the nuclear family all constitute social groups whose significance for the communication of psychopathology and deviant behaviour is only now beginning to come under systematic study. Apart from the difficulties of defining and observing such key groups, there remains the major problem of measuring the social forces which operate within and upon any given group. This problem can be approached in a number of ways: attention can be focussed upon the social functioning of individuals, or upon relationships between individuals; on relatively objective data such as the frequency of events, or on highly subjective feelings and attitudes; on the direct rating of informants' accounts, or on judgments and interpretations made by interviewers. Recent work in this field has been concerned largely with questions of validity and reliability, particularly of the measurement of family relationships.

To investigate the social functioning of psychiatric patients in the community, one research group (76) has constructed a standard social interview which pays regard to housing conditions, employment, family income level, marital adjustment, child management, and personal interaction with other members of the household and immediate social orbit. Each item is rated on a 4-point scale ranging from 0 ("satisfactory, no difficulties") to 3 ("severe difficulties or dissatisfaction") , and assigned to one of three principal categories:

1. *Material conditions:* comprising factual data on housing conditions, family income and situational handicaps (including chronic physical illness and disability) ;
2. *Management and competence:* as shown by the individual's ability to conduct his social life and personal relationships, e.g. standards of marital adjustment and interaction with relatives and neighbors;
3. *Role satisfaction:* as judged from the individual's expressed attitudes to living conditions, occupation and social role, e.g. as housewife, parent, retired person.

The item -ratings are summarized in Table XXXVII.

This interview is intended to be administered to men and women in a wide range of social circumstances: married or single, with or without children; living alone or in a household group. The appropriate items are rated in each case, any not applicable being omitted. The method requires that, if the patient is a member of a family or household group, a key informant (usually the

TABLE XXXVII

CLASSIFICATION OF SOCIAL ADJUSTMENT RATINGS

Material Conditions	Management and Competence	Patient's Satisfaction
Housing conditions	Household care	with house and district
—	Occupational stability	(with employment (with social role
Household income	Management of money	with financial state
—	Marital adjustment	—
Situational handicaps to:	Standard (and extent) of:	
Leisure and social activities		with leisure and social activities
Interaction with relatives		
Interaction with workmates		
Interaction with neighbours		
Child management		with parental role

Source: Cooper *et al.* (76).

spouse) shall also be present at interview. It also demands that for comparative studies each group shall be matched, not only by age, sex and social class, but by all variables which determine the items to be rated. Thus, a housewife with children at home cannot be matched with a married woman who has no children; nor with one who employs a child-minder or goes out to work. The sampling frame must, therefore, provide access to the demographic and social data necessary for detailed matching.

In a study of chronic neurotic illness, index patients from a general practice population were compared with controls drawn from the same practice lists (76). Members of both groups had a standard clinical interview (148) which clearly differentiated "cases" and "normals." Comparison of the two groups on the social interview ratings showed strong associations between the clinical state and all aspects of social adjustment, especially those grouped under social competence and role satisfaction. These findings, as is usual in cross-sectional surveys, tell us nothing about the underlying causal relationships; they do, however, provide the necessary base-line for longitudinal and evaluative studies.

Any global assessment of social functioning must inevitably

be superficial; more intensive studies are needed of those aspects which appear to have special relevance to mental health and illness. A case in point is marital adjustment, which is notoriously difficult to assess reliably after a single interview. One fairly objective measure is the time-budget, which comprises a record of the activities of both spouses during a limited period of time. Kreitman and his co-workers have recently reported the use of this technique in a controlled study of marital interaction and neurosis (253, 344). Activities over the seven days prior to interview were charted for each individual, and the two groups then compared in terms of the total amount of time spent together. The results, summarized in Table XXXVIII, showed that men in the neurotic group spent significantly more time alone with their wives than did those in the control group.

TABLE XXXVIII
TIME ALLOCATION OF NEUROTIC AND NORMAL HUSBANDS AND
THEIR WIVES: MEAN VALUES†

	Neurotic Husbands and Their Wives ($n = 76$)	*Normal Husbands and Their Wives* ($n = 44$)	*Differ- ence*
(a) Spouses together: *without others*			
in the same room	33.6	27.6	6.0*
in different room	8.2	7.0	1.2
outside the home	3.5	2.9	0.6
Total	45.4	37.3	8.1*
with others Total	13.7	13.9	— 0.2
Total time spouses together	59.1	51.2	7.9*
(b) Spouses apart	8.7	7.8	0.9

*P <0.05
†time potentially shareable (i.e. outside working hours) during seven-day period
Source: Nelson *et al.* (344).

The findings are open to more than one interpretation, being consistent either with the view that neurotic concordance in married couples is due to assortative mating (432), or with the opposing belief that it can be ascribed to pathogenic interaction and imitative modelling (252). Two concomitant findings favoured the latter hypothesis; namely, that with the duration of marriage the level of neurotic symptoms among the index patients' wives appeared to rise, and conversely that the level of their outside social contacts appeared to fall.

A more direct assault on the problem of measuring family relationships has been described by Brown and Rutter (45), who have also comprehensively reviewed the literature on this subject (410). The technique they evolved is complex and time-consuming, but carries the advantage of permitting subjective information to be rated reliably. Briefly, they used two types of scale for measuring feeling and emotion: one was simply a count of the negative and positive statements made by a respondent during interview about his spouse and children, individually. The other was an overall assessment which took into account such nuances as the respondent's tone of voice. Thus, the feelings of a patient's wife towards him was judged in terms of the warmth and sympathy with which she spoke of his symptoms and handicaps.

A study of joint interviews with thirty families indicated that ratings of this type could be made with surprisingly high reliability, provided the interviewers had undergone careful training. On a 6-point scale for emotional warmth, for example, complete agreement between raters was obtained in 52 percent of interviews, and agreement to within one point in a further 35 percent. In general, correlation between the two sets of independent ratings were of the order of +0.80 or higher. With the aid of this technique it should be possible to draw meaningful conclusions about the family relationships of different subgroups in the general population, including those characterized by psychiatric disturbance.

DATA PROCESSING AND ANALYSIS

Undoubtedly, the single most influential development of recent times, for survey research as a whole and for epidemiology in particular, has been the advent of the electronic computer. It is fair to say that the speed and facility with which the computer can process large quantities of data has opened up fresh vistas for the epidemiologist. Nevertheless, enthusiasm for this new research tool must be tempered by an awareness of its practical limitations. Computers are subject to a variety of technical faults, which may reduce their value to the research worker. In the words of Massey (309) :

> To most epidemiologists . . . the computer from, say, 1958-63 was still a box (or a room) full of wires, for which extravagant promises were made, but which typically were out of order when they went to use them. . . . It would be impossible to pretend that these problems are now solved, but today the machine is at least much more likely to be a help than a hindrance.

Furthermore, because the language and operation of computers remains largely a matter for experts, the ordinary medical investigator is compelled to rely upon others for the analysis of his data. The quantity of information may be such that it is difficult for him to detect possible discrepancies by simple inspection of the computer print-out. Under these circumstances, the risk of error is multiplied.

To some extent, the difficulty will be resolved by the increasing accessibility of computers, the simplification of their language, and the growth of standard computer programs which can be adapted to meet the needs of individual projects. Massey has pointed out that the construction of tables, with corresponding percentages, means, standard deviations, correlation coefficients and chi-square values where appropriate, accounts for the bulk of statistical procedures in survey analysis. Analysis of variance and co-variance, multiple regression analysis and principal components analysis together cover most of the remainder. With this degree of stereotyping of research requirements, it should become increasingly feasible for medical investigators with no specialised training to process their own data, using available sets of "package" programs.

Computers have played an important part in some of the developments outlined in earlier sections of this chapter; for example, in the standardizing of diagnostic procedures (436, 473), the automation of multiphasic screening programs (69) and the monitoring of physiological signals (18). Their major contributions, however, have been made in other fields. First, they have influenced methods of data collection, notably through the growth of record linkage systems. Secondly, they have greatly facilitated the use of multivariate techniques of statistical analysis. Finally, they have rendered possible experimental studies which were formerly impracticable, such as the construction and testing of predictive models of disease and medical care. Each of these effects will be considered briefly in relation to psychiatric research.

Record Linkage Systems

Record linkage has been defined as the process of bringing together data recorded at different times and places into a series of personal cumulative files (2). Such a system does not provide new information, but rather makes accessible that which would otherwise be difficult to use because so widely scattered and inaccessible.

The principle is by no means new in epidemiology, where it has been applied on an *ad hoc* basis to many investigations. The best-known instances relate to fatal disease, death registration being one of the few statistical procedures universal in the developed countries. A case in point is the association between mortality from bronchial carcinoma and previously recorded smoking history (95). The same principle has been applied to the study of mortality among psychiatric patients, such as heroin addicts (216) and attempted suicides (458). The linking of mental hospital admission data with birth certification yielded a valuable new perspective on the social mobility of schizophrenic patients (149). In studies of this kind, the investigators have had to amass their material from widely separated sources, at the expense of great effort. The development of linked record systems offers the prospect that in future morbidity data will be related to vital events quite quickly and easily.

The usefulness of record linkage on a national or regional scale will vary greatly, according to the type of information required. Medical data can be roughly categorized into those such as hospital discharge and cause of death, which can be readily enumerated, and those such as clinical notes, radiographs and electrocardiographs, which under ordinary circumstances cannot be enumerated (365). Similarly, demographic and social data comprise vital events (births, marriages, deaths) which are enumerable, and all the lesser events and life-experiences of which no official record is kept, and which are not easily quantified. It follows that the most effective national record linkage will be that which relates hospital in-patient records to circumstances of birth and death. The scope for such a system in psychiatry is limited, especially now that in-patient records yield so incomplete a picture even of the major psychoses.

Extension of record linkage beyond these well-defined boundaries presents a number of problems. The inclusion of out-patient and general practice statistics, for example, would place enormous demands on the recording system, while at the same time lowering the reliability of the data. Extension to non-medical sources, such as prisons, schools and social agencies, would give rise to similar technical difficulties; it would also conflict with medical ethics. Already, there is widespread public misgiving about the central storage of medical and other confidential information in "data banks," and their possible abuse by government or commercial organizations. The medical profession, more than any other section of the community, has to be alert to such dangers.

Three adaptations of record linkage can help to create an effective compromise. First, the area case-register, whose use has been discussed in Chapters 2 and 3, is a local linkage system which can store a great deal of useful information while avoiding the worst features of bureaucratic centralism. Secondly, anterospective cohort studies such as the Berkeley Growth Study (293) and the British Child Health Survey (96) can provide the basis for a continuing linkage of medical, educational and social data about representative population samples within specific age-groups. Finally, a record linkage system can be based on a sample of *doctors*. Thus, in Great Britain the Records and Statistics Unit of the Royal College of General Practitioners monitors weekly returns from some 40 practices, using a special record-card on which morbidity and personal data are entered according to a standard format (307).

The existence of such schemes affords the possibility of a two-tiered system, whereby basic data stored nationally could on occasion be linked with more detailed information stored locally or in a research centre. A project of this kind would permit the retrieval of data about persons who had moved outside the limits of an area register, or who had been lost from a cohort study.

Techniques of Multivariate Analysis

An increasingly frequent situation in psychiatric research is that in which a number of independent observers are asked to make ratings on the same group of subjects, with a view to establishing the reliability of observer judgments. In some instances, quite simple measures of agreement can be employed: if, for example, each item is scored either "1" or "0" according to whether it is judged to be present or absent (312). More often, each item has to be scored on a rating-scale with a number of points; provided certain conditions obtain, the appropriate test is then a two-way or three-way analysis of variance. This technique allows the total variation in a set of data to be divided into components, each associated with a source of variation whose relative importance can thus be assessed.

A convenient example is provided by a study in which five psychiatrists examined a total of forty hospital patients, in order to test the reliability of a standardized interview technique (148). Each patient was seen by two raters, one of whom administered the interview while the other acted as a co-rater. The patients were randomly assigned to pairs of raters, and within the pairs, each psychiatrist acted twice as interviewer and twice as co-rater. In the course of the standardized interview, twenty-two items were rated, covering a wide range of reported symptoms and abnormal behaviour. In addition to product-moment correlation and the value of "weighted kappa" (112) for each item, the results were expressed as a three-way analysis of variance, as in Table XXXIX.

When the mean square values for the three main variables—doctors, patients and clinical items—were tested against that for the residual variance it was found that the mean squares for patients and items were significant at the 0.01 level, while the mean square for doctors was not: in other words, there was no significant

TABLE XXXIX
RELIABILITY OF A STANDARDIZED PSYCHIATRIC INTERVIEW:
RESULTS OF THREE-WAY ANALYSIS OF VARIANCE

	SSq.	d.f.	MSq.
Source of Variations			
Between patients	83.54	39	2.14†
Between items	74.47	19	3.92†
Between doctors	0.12	1	0.12 NS
Interactions			
Patients × items	259.37	741	0.35*
Patients × doctors	3.50	39	0.09 NS
Items × doctors	2.10	19	0.11 NS
Residual			
Patients × doctors × items	148.52	741	0.20
Total	571.61	1599	

†Significant at 0.01 level
*Significant at 0.05 level
Source: Goldberg *et al.* (148).

variation between interviewer and co-rater. The low mean square values for interaction between doctors and items, and between doctors and patients, indicate that the doctors' rating standards remained consistent from one item to the next and from one patient to the next.

In the analysis of complex survey data, computers enable the effects of numbers of independent variables to be examined simultaneously. This approach represents a great advance over the older techniques in which each of a series of variables was examined consecutively, particularly since it was not then as a rule feasible to standardize for any basic demographic variables other than age and sex. The value of multiple regression analysis is perhaps more apparent where a number of determinants of disease are competing for research priority. In the Framingham survey, for example, this technique was used to assess the relative weights to be given age, body weight, systolic blood-pressure, serum cholesterol level, haemoglobin concentration, electrocardiogram, and smoking habits as predictors of ischaemic heart disease (456).

In psychiatry, causal factors cannot yet be so nicely quantified, although an essentially similar approach is now being adopted in studying the ecology of suicide and attempted suicide (13, 53). Multiple regression analysis can already help to explain the observed variation in reported prevalence rates, and in the utilization of psychiatric services. Thus, a survey of psychiatric illness in nearly fifty general practices (423) yielded one-year total prevalence rates ranging from 38 to 323 per 1,000 adults at risk. The single index found to have highest correlation with the psychiatric rates was that of patient mobility. Addition of an index of social class distribution did not add significantly to the multiple correlation; since this second index was highly correlated with the first, both were "explaining" the same part of the total variance. The correlation coefficient obtained from this regression was +0.58 ($r^2 = 0.34$); in other words, demographic differences in the practice populations accounted for about one-third of the total variance in reported morbidity.

The influence of the doctors' attitudes and diagnostic habits had been examined by means of a standardized questionnaire. When the resulting attitude scores were included in a regression analysis with the demographic data, they gave a multiple correlation of +0.69 ($r^2 = 0.48$), accounting for half the total nonrandom variance. Thus, both demographic and attitudinal factors were important causes of the variation in reported prevalence rates.

Another statistical problem with increasing implications for psychiatric research is that of testing for possible *clustering* of individuals or units. The term "cluster" is used in two senses which should be distinguished. First, it can relate literally to the incidence of a disease in space and time. In this context, statistical methods are employed to test the epidemicity of a given disease which may or may not be of infective origin: two such techniques, for example, have been developed and applied in research on acute leukaemia (87, 106). The suggestion that Down's syndrome (mongolism) might be due to an infective agent, such as the virus of infective hepatitis (248, 444), has encouraged a number of workers to look for time-and-space clustering in mongol births.

Secondly, "cluster" is used to denote a type of statistical analysis concerned with the grouping of units in vector space: as such it has been applied to problems in the classification of psychiatric patients (311), and has obvious relevance to the general issue of the delineation of syndromes. Techniques of cluster analysis may help to delimit population sub-groups, homogeneous in certain respects, which are of interest in survey research. For example, it has been a long-standing difficulty of ecological surveys that the official administrative boundaries such as precincts, wards and arrondisements correspond roughly at best to socio-cultural units. With the aid of suitable computer programs, it is now possible to identify clusters of small census tracts which are homogeneous in socio-cultural terms, and whose morbidity rates can be more meaningfully compared. This point is demonstrated by a study of referral to an urban Child Guidance Clinic (135). Analysis of the referral rates for twenty electoral wards disclosed associations with a number of socio-economic indices, including social class distribution and proportion of owner-occupied dwellings. Since each electoral ward was a relatively large heterogeneous unit of about 15,000 persons in widely varying social circumstances, the wards were broken down into their constituent enumeration districts and re-combined into more homogeneous socio-economic units by means of a cluster analysis. Table XL summarizes the results of this exercise, showing how the ecological correlations were strengthened.

TABLE XL
CORRELATION OF CHILD GUIDANCE REFERRAL RATES WITH DEMOGRAPHIC AND SOCIOECONOMIC INDICES

Index	*Electoral Wards* *(n = 20)*	*Enumeration District Clusters* *(n = 22)*
Proportion foreign-born residents	+0.064	+0.278
Migration rate	—0.222	—0.098
Proportion Social Classes I and II	—0.338	—0.649
Proportion Social Classes IV and V	+0.371	+0.670
Proportion owner-occupiers	—0.617	—0.569
Density of population	+0.413	+0.679
Proportion sharing dwelling	+0.162	+0.006

Source: Gath *et al.* (135) and unpublished data

Modelling and Simulation

So far, few attempts have been made to study the behaviour of mental disorders in populations by means of predictive models. In other fields of epidemiology, this approach has received more attention, particularly with regard to infectious disease. Any such model translates into mathematical terms the classification of a given population into, say, infective, susceptible and immune persons, and is designed to forecast changes in the number and composition of each class under certain circumstances. In order to do so, it has to make assumptions about the contacts which will occur within the population, and the conditions necessary for disease transmission. It must also presuppose either that relevant events are pre-determined, or else that they occur to some extent randomly. The mathematical principles, which are outside the scope of this summary, are now well established (15, 232).

It has long been recognized that mathematical models are potentially valuable in explaining the behaviour and spread of diseases within communities. The computer's special contribution has been to make feasible the testing of relatively complex models which, insofar as they can take into account large numbers of relevant variables, approximate to the conditions of a real epidemic. Where the mode of transmission is well understood, all the relevant variables may be quantified and introduced into the equations for the model. Thus, in the study of malaria, such parameters as the anopheline density, the proportion of infective mosquitoes, the time taken for completion of the parasite's lifecycle, the proportion of the human population receiving inocula, and the incubation interval have been used (292). Corresponding models can be constructed for other host-borne diseases. They serve as useful guides to the planning of preventive programmes, and for comparison of the cost-effectiveness of alternative preventive measures (337).

The extension of this approach to non-infectious diseases has been on too small a scale to permit any firm assessment of its potential. The incidence of industrial accidents has been subjected to repeated mathematical analysis since it was shown over 50 years ago that the observed frequency distribution was best fitted by a model of unequal accident liability (166). More recently, stochastic models have begun to be applied to the study of remittent diseases such as rheumatoid arthritis (21, 66).

In psychiatry, model-building is an only too-familiar exercise in relation to the physiological and psychological mechanisms underlying the clinical picture. Mathematical models, however, have been employed almost exclusively by geneticists confronted by frequency distributions which do not conform to simple Mendelian laws. Slater (431), for example, put forward a monogenic theory of schizophrenia, according to which the disorder manifests itself in all homozygotes and also in a proportion of heterozygotes. Given an expectancy of 0.8 percent for the general population, it was possible to estimate the proportion of heterozygotes which would have to manifest the disease for different gene frequencies. By comparing the observed frequency for the sibs and children of schizophrenic patients, Slater found close correspondence with a model based on an estimated gene frequency of 0.015, and a manifestation rate among heterozygotes of 26 percent. This type of model is of restricted utility, since the factors determining gene penetrance remain unexplained. Furthermore, the reliability of the diagnostic and epidemiological data can be called in question.

Similar objections can be raised to studies of the major functional psychoses which rest on the hypothesis that they are essentially auto-immune diseases. Burch (54) has claimed that the age-specific incidence of both schizophrenia and manic-depressive psychosis are in keeping with this hypothesis. Since, however, his incidence rates were derived from hospital first-admission statistics, which cannot be accepted as a measure of inception, the whole basis for this argument is shaky.

A more limited, but in some ways more satisfactory, application of modelling is the kind of computer exercise in which the behaviour of a disorder in a given population is simulated repeatedly, in order to test the accuracy of different factor weightings. Such an exercise was undertaken by Kreitman and his co-workers in their study of attempted suicide in Edinburgh (254).

Finally, Markovian planning models can be used to predict

future demands for mental health services, as well as future changes in the available resources under specified conditions. An application of Markov processes to epidemiological psychiatry was reported as far back as the mid-1950s (308), but the scope of this method has been greatly enlarged by modern computer techniques (343).

FUTURE PROSPECTS

This brief review of current advances in survey method leads naturally to a consideration of the future development of epidemiological psychiatry. Improvements in technique, it is safe to assume, will not affect the broad principles of research strategy and design, outlined in Chapter 2; nor is the scope of their application, as set out in the next three chapters, likely to undergo any radical alteration. Equally, the fundamental problems of psychiatry can be expected to remain constant, though they may be reformulated in somewhat different terms. No doubt, as patterns of morbidity in the general population continue to change, some major public health issues of our day will recede in importance, while others come to the forefront. Senile and presenile degenerative disorders, drug dependence of various types, and the neuropsychiatric syndromes associated with head injury, are examples of categories which seem destined to gain in prominence as subjects for epidemiological enquiry. But these will be changes in emphasis, rather than in direction.

What may be significantly modified is the extent to which such research activities continue to be regarded as part of a distinct, specialized discipline. Infectious epidemiology from its early days has been characterized by a close linkage between field-survey and laboratory investigations. Non-infectious epidemiology has grown up more recently, as one aspect of an approach to the prevention of disease which also incorporates clinical and laboratory techniques. In short, epidemiology today forms an integral part of the scientific basis of preventive medicine.

Similar trends can be discerned in the field of mental health, where survey methods are now accepted as a basic part of their armoury by workers studying problems of genetics, mental retardation, the behaviour disorders of childhood, alcoholism and drug addiction. In these and other areas of psychiatric research, the main aim of epidemiology is to provide a rational basis for preventive action. As yet, however, the concept of prevention of mental disorders represents little more than an ideal.

Given the present limitations of knowledge, any realistic programme of prevention in psychiatry must concentrate heavily on the secondary and tertiary stages; that is to say, on the early recognition and treatment of established disease, and the reduction of chronic handicaps. In this context, epidemiological methods have a vital part to play in the assessment of service needs, the operational study of existing services and the evaluation of experimental schemes. It may be, indeed, that the field of operational and evaluative studies of services will afford the greatest scope for epidemiological psychiatry during the next one or two decades.

To what extent the ultimate goal of primary prevention will prove attainable, and how closely it can be approached through specific measures based on a knowledge of causation, must be a matter for conjecture. Experience in other branches of medicine leads us to expect that even where specific aetiological factors are discovered, as in the relationship between bronchial carcinoma and cigarette smoking, major obstacles to prevention will still have to be overcome. Insofar as the causes of mental disorder lie buried at the roots of our society, the development of preventive psychiatry must attend, not only on scientific advance, but upon a complex process of political, economic and socio-cultural change. It must be said that observation of current political and social trends leaves few grounds for easy optimism.

From this standpoint, the long-term future of epidemiological research in psychiatry can be seen to rest, less with technological progress than with the growth of a philosophy of medicine which views the sickness of individuals in relation to the health of communities, and regards disease prevention as perhaps the single most important field for the application of scientific methods to humanitarian ends.

REFERENCES

1. Abey-Wickrama, I., A'Brook, M.F., Gattoni, F.E.G. and Herridge, C.F. (1969) : Mental hospital admissions and aircraft noise. *Lancet, 2:* 1275.

2. Acheson, E.D. (1967): *Medical Record Linkage.* London, O.U.P. for the Nuffield Provincial Hospitals Trust.

3. Ackner, B. (1960): Emotional aspects of hysterectomy. A follow-up of 50 patients under the age of 40. *Adv Psychosom Med (Basel); 1:* 248.

4. Adelstein, A.M., Downham, D.Y., Stein, Z. and Susser, M.W. (1968): The epidemiology of mental illness in an English city. *Soc Psychiatry, 3:* 47.

5. Ahrenfeldt, R.H. (1958): *Psychiatry in the British Army in the Second World War.* London, Routledge and Kegan Paul.

6. Alarcon, R. de (1969): The spread of heroin abuse in a community. *WHO Bulletin on Narcotics, 21:* 17.

7. Alarcon, R. de and Rathod, N.H. (1968): Prevalence and early detection of heroin abuse. *Br Med J, 2:* 549.

8. Allan, F.N. and Kaufman, N. (1948): Nervous factors in general practice. *JAMA, 138:* 1135.

9. American Psychiatric Association (1968): *Diagnostic and Statistical Manual of Mental Disorders,* 2nd ed. Washington, A.P.A.

10. Anderson, V.E. (1964) : Genetics. In Stevens, H.A. and Heber, R. (Eds.): *Mental Retardation: A Review of Research.* Chicago & London, University of Chicago Press.

11. Astrup, C. and Ødegaard, Ø. (1960): The influence of hospital facilities and other local factors upon admission to psychiatric hospitals. *Acta Psychiat Scand, 35:* 289.

12. Bagley, C. (1968): The evaluation of a suicide prevention scheme by an ecological method. *Soc Sci Med, 2:* 1.

13. Bagley, C. and Greer, S. (1971): Clinical and social predictors of repeated attempted suicide: a multivariate analysis. *Br J Psychiatry, 119:* 515.

14. Bahn, A.K., Gardner, E.A., Alltop, L., Knalterud, G.K. and Solomon, M. (1966): Admission and prevalence rates for psychiatric facilities in four Register areas. *Am J Public Health, 56:* 2033.

15. Bailey, N.T.J. (1967): The simulation of stochastic epidemics in two dimensions. Proc. 5th Berkeley Symp Math Statist Probab, *4:* 237.

16. Bannister, D. (1968): The logical requirements of research into schizophrenia. *Br J Psychiatry, 114:* 181.

17. Barker, M.G. (1968): Psychiatric illness after hysterectomy. *Br Med J, 1:* 91.
18. Barnett, G.O. (1968): Computers in patient care. *N Engl J Med, 279:* 1321.
19. Barraclough, B.M. (1971): Personal communication.
20. Barraclough, B.M. and Shea, N. (1970): Suicide and Samaritan clients. *Lancet, 2:* 868.
21. Beall, G. and Cobb, S. (1961): The frequency distribution of episodes of rheumatoid arthritis as shown by periodic examination. *J Chronic Dis, 14:* 291.
22. Belknap, I. (1956): *Human Problems of a State Mental Hospital.* New York, McGraw Hill.
23. Belknap, I. and Jaco, E.G. (1953): The epidemiology of mental disorders in a political-type city, 1946-52. In *Inter-relations Between the Social Environment and Psychiatric Disorders.* New York, Milbank Memorial Fund.
24. Bell, Luther V. (1844): *26th Annual Report of the McLean Asylum for the Insane, 1843,* p. 28. James Loring Press.
25. Bennet, G. (1970): Bristol Floods 1968. A controlled survey of the effects of a local community disaster. *Br Med J, 3:* 454.
26. Bennett, D.H., Folkard, S. and Nicholson, A.K. (1961): Resettlement unit in a mental hospital. *Lancet, 2:* 539.
27. Bingham, W.V. (1946): Inequalities in adult capacity—from military data. *Science, 104:* 147.
28. Blum, R.H. (1962): Case identification in psychiatric epidemiology: methods and problems. *Milbank Mem Fund Q, 40:* 253.
29. Böök, J.A. (1953): A genetic and neuropsychiatric investigation of a North Swedish population. *Acta Genet (Basel), 4:* 1.
30. Borkenstein, R.F., Crowther, R.F., Shumate, R.P., Ziel, W.B., Zylman, R. (Dale, A., Ed.) (1964): *The Role of the Drinking Driver in Traffic Accidents.* Bloomington, Indiana University, Dept. of Police Administration.
31. Bott, E. (1957): *Family and Social Network.* London, Tavistock.
32. Bourdillon, R.E., Clark, C.A., Ridges, A.P., Sheppard, P.M., Harper, P. and Leslie, S.A. (1965): Pink spot in the urine of schizophrenics. *Nature, 208:* 453.
33. Bourne, P.G., Rose, R.M. and Mason, J.W. (1967): Urinary 17-hydroxy-corticosteroid levels: Data on seven helicopter ambulance medics in combat. *Arch Gen Psychiatry, 17:* 104.
34. Bowlby, J. (1951): *Maternal care and mental health. WHO Monograph Series, No. 2.* Geneva, WHO.
35. Bowlby, J. (1962): Childhood bereavement and psychiatric illness. In Richter, D., Tanner, J.M., Taylor, Lord, and Zangwill, O.L. (Eds.):

Aspects of Psychiatric Research. London, Oxford University Press, p. 264.

36. Brandon, S. and Gruenberg, E.M. (1966): Measurement of the incidence of chronic severe social breakdown syndrome. In Evaluating the Effectiveness of Mental Health Services. *Milbank Mem Fund Q, 44:* 129.

37. Bremer, J. (1951): Social psychiatric investigation of a small community in Northern Norway. *Acta Psychiatr Neurol Scand, (Suppl. 62).*

38. Epidemiology of non-communicable disease. *Br Med Bull, 27 (No. 1).* London, The British Council.

39. Brodman, K., Erdmann, A.J., Lorge, I., Wolff, H.G. and Broadbent, T.H. (1952): The Cornell Medical Index Health Questionnaire III. The evaluation of emotional disturbances. *J Clin Psychol, 8:* 119.

40. Brooke, E.M. (1959): National statistics in the epidemiology of mental illness. *J Ment Sci, 105:* 893.

41. Brown, A.C. (1965): The general morbidity of neurotic patients. Cambridge University M.D. thesis. Unpublished.

42. Brown, G.W. and Birley, J.L.T. (1968): Crises and life changes and the onset of schizophrenia. *J Health Soc Behav, 9:* 203.

43. Brown, G.W., Carstairs, G.M. and Topping, G. (1958): Post-hospital adjustment of chronic mental patients. *Lancet, 2:* 685.

44. Brown, G.W., Monck, E.M., Carstairs, G.M. and Wing, J.K. (1962): Influence of family life on the course of schizophrenic illness. *Br J Prev Soc Med, 16:* 55.

45. Brown, G.W. and Rutter, M. (1966): The measurement of family activities and relationships: a methodological study. *Human Relations, 19:* 241.

46. Brugger, C. (1933): Psychiatrische Ergebnisse einer medizinischen, anthropologischen, und soziologischen bevölkerungsuntersuchung. *Z Neur, 146:* 489.

47. Bruhn, J.G. (1962). Broken homes among attempted suicides and psychiatric out-patients: a comparative study. *J Ment Sci, 108:* 772.

48. Bryson, E. (1945): The psychosomatic approach in gynaecological practice. *Practitioner, 155:* 378.

49. Buck, C.W. and Hobbs, G.E. (1959). The problem of specificity in psychosomatic illness. *J Psychosom Res, 3:* 227.

50. Buck, C.W. and Laughton, K.B. (1959) : Family patterns of illness: the effect of psychoneurosis in the parent upon illness in the child. *Acta Psychiatr Scand, 34:* 165.

51. Buck, R.W. (1930): *Bull Mass Soc Ment Hyg, 60:* 2.

52. Bucknill, J.C. and Tuke, D.H. (1874): *A Manual of Psychological Medicine.* Containing the lunacy laws, the nosology, aetiology, statistics, description, diagnosis, pathology and treatment of insanity with appendix of cases. London, Churchill.

55. Burnet, Sir MacFarlane (1962): *Natural History of Infectious Disease.* tion of parasuicide ("attempted suicide") rates in Edinburgh. *Br J Prev Soc Med, 24:* 182.

54. Burch, P.R.J. (1964) : Manic-depressive psychosis: some new aetiological considerations. *Br J Psychiatry, 110:* 808.

55. Burnet, Sir MacFarlane (1962) : *Natural History of Infectious Disease.* Cambridge University Press.

56. Burt, C. (1955): *The Subnormal Mind,* 3rd ed. London, Oxford University Press.

57. Carse, J., Panton, N.E. and Watt, A. (1958): A district mental health service: the Worthing experiment. *Lancet, 1:* 39.

58. Casey, M.D., Blank, C.E., Street, D.R.R., Segall, L.J., McDougall, J.H., McGrath, P.J. and Skinner, J.L. (1966): YY chromosomes and antisocial behaviour. *Lancet, 2:* 859.

59. Castell, J.H.F. and Mittler, P.J. (1965): Intelligence of patients in subnormality hospitals: a survey of admissions in 1961. *Br J Psychiatry, 111:* 219.

60. Cattell, R.B. (1957): *Sixteen Personality Factor Questionnaire (revised edition).* Institute for Personality and Ability Testing, Champaign, Illinois.

61. Cattell, R.B. (1965) : *The Scientific Analysis of Personality.* Pelican Books No. A712. Harmondsworth, Middlesex, Penguin Books.

62. Cavan, R.S. (1928): *Suicide.* Chicago, University of Chicago Press.

63. Central Health Services Council (1956): *Report of the sub-committee on the medical care of epileptics* (Cohen Committee). London, H.M.S.O.

64. Champion, Y. (1958): *Migration et maladie mentale.* Paris, Librairie Arnette.

65. Clark, R.E. (1949): Psychosis, income and occupational prestige. *Am J Sociol, 54:* 433.

66. Cobb, S. (1962): A method for the epidemiologic study of remittent disease. *Am J Public Health, 52:* 1119.

67. Cohen, B.H., Lilienfeld, A.M. and Sigler, A.T. (1963): Some epidemiological aspects of 'mongolism': a review. *Am J Public Health, 53:* 223.

68. Cohen, B.M. and Fairbank, R. (1938): Statistical contributions from the Mental Hygiene Study of the Eastern Health District of Baltimore II: Psychosis in the E.H.D. in 1933. *Am J Psychiatry, 94:* 1377.

69. Collen, M.F., Rubin, L., Neyman, J., Dantzig, G.B., Baer, R.M. and Siegelaub, A.B. (1964): Automated multiphasic screening and diagnosis. *Am J Public Health, 54:* 741.

70. Commission on Chronic Illness (1957): *Prevention of Chronic Illness. Chronic Illness in the United States, Vol. 1.* Cambridge, Mass., Harvard University Press for the Commonwealth Fund.

71. Commonwealth Fund (1936) : *Snow on Cholera.* New York, The Commonwealth Fund. London, Oxford University Press.

72. Cook, T., Morgan, H.G. and Pollak, B. (1968): The Rathcoole experiment: first year at a hostel for vagrant alcoholics. *Br Med J, 1:* 240.
73. Cooper, B. (1961): Social class and prognosis in schizophrenia. *Br J Prev Soc Med, 15:* 17.
74. Cooper, B. (1964): The epidemiological approach to psychosomatic medicine. *J Psychosom Res, 8:* 9.
75. Cooper, B. (1966): Psychiatric disorder in hospital and general practice. *Soc Psychiatry, 1:* 7.
76. Cooper, B., Eastwood, M.R. and Sylph, J. (1970): Psychiatric morbidity and social adjustment in a general practice population. In: Hare, E.H. and Wing, J.K.: *Psychiatric Epidemiology*. London and New York, Oxford University Press.
77. Cooper, B., Fry, J. and Kalton, G. (1969): A longitudinal study of psychiatric morbidity in a general practice population. *Br J Prev Soc Med, 23:* 210.
78. Cooper, B. and Shepherd, M. (1970): Life change, stress and mental disorder: the ecological approach In Price, J.H. (Ed.): *Modern Trends in Psychological Medicine*. London, Butterworth.
79. Cooper, B. and Shepherd, M. (1972): Epidemiology and abnormal psychology In Eysenck, H.J. (Ed.): *Handbook of Abnormal Psychology*, 2nd ed. London, Pitman (in press).
80. Cooper, J.E., Kendell, R.E., Gurland, B.J. and Sartorius, N. (1969): Cross-national study of diagnosis of mental disorders: Some results from the first comparative investigation. *Am J Psychiatry, 125 (Suppl.,* April issue).
81. Court-Brown, W.M. (1967): Human population cytogenetics. In Neuberger, A. and Tatum, E.L. (Eds.): *Frontiers of Biology*. North-Holland Research Monographs. Amsterdam, North-Holland, Vol. 5.
82. Court-Brown, W.M., Buckton, K.E., Jacobs, P.A., Tough, I.M., Kuenssberg, E.V. and Knox, J.D.E. (1966): Study of a group of adults randomly selected from the list of several general practitioners. Chromosome studies on adults. Eugenic Laboratory Memoirs, Series XLII, the Galton Laboratory. London, Cambridge University Press.
83. Crown, S. and Crisp, A.H. (1966): A short clinical diagnostic self-rating scale for psychoneurotic patients. *Br J Psychiatry, 112:* 917.
84. Crown, S., Duncan, K.P. and Howell, R.W. (1970): Further evaluation of the Middlesex Hospital Questionnaire (M.H.Q.). *Br. J. Psychiatry, 116:* 33.
85. Culpan, R.H., Davies, B.M. and Oppenheim, A.N. (1960): Incidence of psychiatric illness among hospital out-patients: an application of the Cornell Medical Index. *Br. Med J, 1:* 855.
86. Davenport, C.B. and Muncey, E.B. (1916): Huntington's Chorea in relation to heredity and eugenics. *Am J Insan, 73:* 195.

87. David, F.N. and Barton, D.E. (1966): Two space-time interaction tests for epidemicity. *Br J Prev Soc Med, 20:* 44.
88. Davies, B.E. (1964): Psychiatric illness at general hospital clinics. *Postgrad Med J, 40:* 15.
89. Dawson, R.E., Webster, J.E. and Gurdjian, E.S. (1951): Serial electro-encephalography in acute head injuries. *J Neurosurg, 8:* 613.
90. Dayton, N.A. (1940): *New Facts on Mental Disorders.* Springfield, Thomas.
91. Denmark, J.C. and Eldridge, R.W. (1969): Psychiatric services for the deaf. *Lancet, 2:* 259.
92. Dennehey, C.M. (1966): Childhood bereavement and psychiatric illness. *Br J Psychiatry, 112:* 1049.
93. Dingle, J.H., Badger, G.F., Feller, A.E., Hodges, R.G., Jordan, W.S. and Rammelkamp, C.H. (1956): A study of illness in a group of Cleveland families. *Am J Hyg, 64:* 349.
94. Dohrenwend, B.P. and Dohrenwend, B.S. (1969): Social status and psychological disorder: a causal enquiry. New York, Wiley.
95. Doll, R. and Hill, A.B. (1964). Mortality in relation to smoking: ten years' observations of British doctors. *Br Med J, 1:* 1399.
96. Douglas, J.W.B. (1964): *The Home and the School.* London, Mac-Gibbon and Kee.
97. Douglas, J.W.B. and Blomfield, J.M. (1958) : *Children Under Five: the results of a national survey.* London, Allen and Unwin.
98. Downes, J. and Simon, K. (1954): Characteristics of psychoneurotic patients and their families as revealed in a general morbidity study. *Milbank Mem Fund Q, 32:* 42.
99. Drillien, C.M. (1958): A longitudinal study of the growth and development of prematurely and maturely born children. I. Introduction. *Arch Dis Child, 33:* 417.
100. Drillien, C.M. (1959): A longitudinal study of the growth and development of prematurely and maturely born children. III. Mental development. *Arch Dis Child, 34:* 37.
101. Dunham, H.W. (1965): Social class and schizophrenia. *Am J Orthopsychiatry, 34:* 634.
102. Durkheim, E. (1951) : *Suicide: a study in sociology* (Trans. Spaulding, J.A. and Simpson, G.). Glencoe, Illinois, Free Press.
103. Eastwood, M.R. (1970): Psychiatric morbidity and physical state in a general practice population. In Hare, E.H. and Wing, J.K. (Eds.): *Psychiatric Epidemiology.* London and New York, Oxford University Press.
104. Eastwood, M.R. (1971): Screening for psychiatric disorder. *Psychol Med, 1:* 197.
105. Eaton, J.W. and Weil, R.J. (1955): *Culture and Mental Disorders.* Glencoe, Illinois, Free Press.

106. Ederer, F., Myers, M.H. and Mantel, N. (1964): A statistical problem in space and time: do leukemia cases come in clusters? *Biometrics, 20:* 626.
107. Edwards, G., Williamson, V., Hawker, A., Hensman, C. and Postoyan, S. (1968): Census of a Reception Centre. *Br J Psychiatry, 114,* 1031.
108. Edwin, E., Holten, K., Norum, K.R., Schrumf, A. and Skaug, O.E. (1965): Vitamin B_{12} hypovitaminosis in mental diseases. *Acta Med Scand, 177:* 689.
109. Eitinger, L. (1959): The incidence of mental disease among refugees in Norway. *J Ment Sci, 105:* 326.
110. Esquirol, E. (1838): *Des Maladies Mentales.* Paris, J.B. Bailliere, Libraire de l'Academie Royale de Medecin, vol. 2, p. 723.
111. Essen-Möller, E. (1956) : Individual traits and morbidity in a Swedish rural population. *Acta Psychiatr Scand, (Suppl. 100).*
112. Everitt, B.S. (1968). Moments of the statistics kappa and weighted kappa. *Br J Math Stat Psychol, 21:* 97.
113. Eysenck, H.J. (1952): *Scientific Study of Personality.* London, Routledge & Kegan Paul.
114. Eysenck, H.J. and Eysenck, S.B.G. (1964): *Manual of the Eysenck Personality Inventory.* London, University of London Press.
115. Faergeman, P.M. (1963): *Psychogenic psychoses: a description and follow-up of psychoses following psychological stress.* London, Butterworth.
116. Faris, R.E.L. and Dunham, H.W. (1939). *Mental disorders in urban areas: an ecological study of schizophrenia and other psychoses.* Chicago, University of Chicago Press.
117. Farr, William (1841). Report on the Mortality of Lunatics. *Roy Stat Soc J, 4,* 17.
118. Fenz, W.D. and Epstein, S. (1967): Gradients of physiological arousal in parachutists as a function of an approaching jump. *Psychosom Med, 29:* 33.
119. Fink, R., Goldensohn, S.S., Shapiro, S. and Daily, E. (1967): Treatment of patients designated by family doctors as having emotional problems. *Am J Public Health, 57:* 1550.
120. Fish, F.J. (1960): Senile schizophrenia. *J Ment Sci, 106:* 938.
121. Fletcher, C.M. and Oldham, P.D. (1959): Diagnosis in group research In: Witts, L.J. (Ed.): *Medical Surveys and Clinical Trials.* London, Oxford University Press.
122. Forssman, H. (1970): The mental implications of sex chromosome aberrations. *Br J Psychiatry, 117:* 353.
123. Foulds, G.A. (1965): *Personality and Personal Illness.* London, Tavistock.
124. Fox, R. (1962): Help for the despairing: the work of the Samaritans. *Lancet, 2:* 1102.

125. Fraser, R. (1947): *The Incidence of Neurosis Amongst Factory Workers.* London, H.M.S.O.
126. Fraser, R.M. (1971): The cost of commotion: an analysis of the psychiatric sequelae of the 1969 Belfast riots. *Br J Psychiatry, 118:* 257.
127. Freeman, H.E. and Simmons, O.G. (1963): *The Mental Patient Comes Home.* New York, Wiley.
128. Fremming, K.H. (1951): *The expectation of mental infirmity in a sample of the Danish population.* Occasional Papers on Eugenics, No. 7. London, Cassell.
129. Freudenberg, R.K. (1967): Theory and practice of the rehabilitation of the psychiatrically disabled. *Psychiatr Q, 41:* 698.
130. Friedhoff, A.J. and Van Winkle, E. (1962): Isolation and characterisation of a compound from the urine of schizophrenics. *Nature, 194:* 897.
131. Friedman, S.B., Mason, J.W. and Hamburg, D.A. (1963): Urinary 17-hydroxycorticosteroid levels in parents of children with neoplastic disease. *Psychosom Med, 25:* 364.
132. Fuller, J.G. (1967): *The Day of St. Anthony's Fire.* London, Hutchinson.
133. Galdston, I. (1957): International psychiatry. *Am J Psychiatry, 114:* 103.
134. Gardner, E.A. (1967): The use of a psychiatric case register in the planning and evaluation of a mental health programme. In *Psych Res Report,* No. 22 (April). Am Psychiatr Assoc.
135. Gath, D., Cooper, B. and Gattoni, F.E.G. (1972): Child guidance and delinquency in a London borough. *Psychol Med 2:* 185.
136. Gathercole, C.E. (1966): I.Q. scores and the problem of classification. *Br J Psychiatry, 112:* 1181.
137. General Register Office (1968): *A Glossary of Mental Disorders.* Studies on Medical and Population Subjects, No. 22. London, H.M.S.O.
138. Gerard, D.L. and Houston, L.G. (1953): Family setting and the social ecology of schizophrenia. *Psychiatr Q, 27:* 90.
139. Gibbens, T.C.N. (1963): *Psychiatric Studies of Borstal Lads.* Maudsley Monographs, No. 11. London, Oxford University Press.
140. Gibson, H.B. and West, D.J. (1970): Social and intellectual handicaps as precursors of early delinquency. *Br J Criminol, 10:* 21.
141. Glass, A.J. and Bernucci, R.J. (Eds.) (1966): *Neuropsychiatry in World War II.* Washington, D.C., Office of the Surgeon General, Dept. of the Army.
142. Glidewell, J.C., Gildea, M.C.L., Domke, H.R. and Kantor, M.B. (1959): Behaviour symptoms in children and adjustment in public school. *Human Organization, 17:* 123.
143. Glueck, S. and Glueck, E.T. (1950): *Unravelling Juvenile Delinquency.* New York, Commonwealth Fund.
144. Glueck, S. and Glueck, E.T. (1959): *Predicting Delinquency and Crime.* Cambridge, Mass., Harvard University Press.
145. Goffman, E. (1961): *Asylums.* New York, Anchor Books, Doubleday.

146. Goldberg, D.P. (1969): The identification and assessment of non-psychotic psychiatric illness by means of a questionnaire. Unpublished D.M. thesis, University of Oxford.

147. Goldberg, D.P. and Blackwell, B. (1970): Psychiatric illness in general practice: a detailed study using a new method of case-identification. *Br Med J, 2:* 439.

148. Goldberg, D.P., Cooper, B., Eastwood, M.R., Kedward, H.B. and Shepherd, M. (1970): A standardized psychiatric interview for use in community surveys. *Br J Prev Soc Med, 24:* 18.

149. Goldberg, E.M. and Morrison, S.L. (1963): Schizophrenia and social class. *Br J Psychiatry, 109:* 785.

150. Goldberger, J. (1914): The etiology of pellagra. The significance of certain epidemiological observations with respect thereto. *Public Health Rep, 29 (No. 26):* 1683.

151. Goldberger, J. (1914): The cause and prevention of pellagra. *Public Health Rep, 29 (No. 37):* 2354.

152. Goldberger, J. (1916): The transmissibility of pellagra. Experimental attempt at transmission to the human subject. *Public Health Rep, 31 (No. 46):* 3159.

153. Goldberger, J., Waring, C.H. and Tanner, W.F. (1923): Pellagra prevention by diet among institutional inmates. *Public Health Rep, 38 (No. 41):* 2361.

154. Goldberger, J., Waring, C.H. and Willets, D.G. (1915): The prevention of pellagra. A test of diet among institutional inmates. *Public Health Rep, 30 (No. 43):* 3117.

155. Goldberger, J. and Wheeler, G.A. (1920): The experimental production of pellagra in human subjects by means of diet. *Hyg Lab Bull, 120:* 7.

156. Goldberger, J., Wheeler, G.A. and Sydenstricker, E. (1920): A study of the relation of diet to pellagra incidence in seven textile-mill communities of South Carolina in 1916. *Public Health Rep, 35 (No. 12):* 648.

157. Goldhammer, H. and Marshall, A. (1953): *Psychosis and Civilisation.* Glencoe, Illinois, Free Press.

158. Goldstein, L.G. (1964): Human variables in traffic accidents. A digest of research. *Traffic Safety Res Rev, 8:* 26.

159. Goodman, N. and Tizard, J. (1962): Prevalence of imbecility and idiocy among children in a metropolitan area. *Br Med J, 1:* 216.

160. Gore, C.P., Jones, K., Taylor, W. and Ward, B. (1964): Needs and beds: A regional census of psychiatric hospital patients. *Lancet, 2:* 457.

161. Grad, J. and Sainsbury, P. (1963): Mental illness and the family. *Lancet, 1:* 544.

162. Grad, J. and Sainsbury, P. (1966): Evaluating the community psychiatric

service in Chichester: results. In: Evaluating the Effectiveness of Mental Health Services. *Milbank Mem Fund Q, 44:* 279.

163. Grandjean, E., Münchinger, R., Turrian, V., Haas, P.A., Knoepfel, H.K. and Rosenmund, H. (1955): Investigation into the effects of exposure to trichlorethylene in mechanical engineering. *Br J Indust Med, 12:* 131.

164. Granville-Grossman, K.L. (1968): The early environment in affective disorders. In Coppen, A. and Walk, A. (Eds.): *Recent Developments in Affective Disorders.* Ashford, Kent, Headley Brothers for R.M.P.A.

165. Graunt, J. (1662): *Natural and political observations mentioned in a following index and made upon the Bills of Mortality.* London, Martin and Co.

166. Greenwood, M. and Woods, H.M. (1919): *Industrial Fatigue Research Board Report No. 4.* London, H.M.S.O.

167. Greer, S. (1964): The relationship between parental loss and attempted suicide. *Br J Psychiatry, 110:* 698.

168. Greer, S. and Cawley, R.H. (1966): *Some Observations on the Natural History of Neurotic Illness. Mervyn Archdale Medical Monograph No. 3.* Sydney, Australian Medical Assoc.

169. Gregory, I. (1965): Retrospective estimates of orphanhood from generation life tables. *Milbank Mem Fund Q, 43:* 323.

170. Griesinger, W. (1867): *Mental Pathology and Therapeutics.* Trans. Robertson, C.L. and Rutherford, J. London, The New Sydenham Society.

171. Gruenberg, E.M. (1957): Socially shared psychopathology. In Leighton, A.H., Clausen, J.A. and Wilson, R.N. (Eds.): *Exploration in Social Psychiatry.* London, Tavistock.

172. Gruenberg, E.M. (1964): Epidemiology. In Stevens, H.A. and Heber, R. (Eds.): *Mental Retardation: a review of research.* Chicago & London, University of Chicago Press.

173. Gruenberg, E.M. (1969): From practice to theory: community mental health services and the nature of psychoses. *Lancet, 1:* 721.

174. Gruenberg, E.M., Brandon, S. and Kasius, R.V. (1966): Identifying cases of the Social Breakdown Syndrome. In: Evaluating the effectiveness of mental health services. *Milbank Mem Fund Q, 44:* 150.

175. Gruenberg, E.M., Snow, H.B. and Bennett, C.L. (1969): Preventing the Social Breakdown Syndrome. In Redlich, F.C. (Ed.): *Social Psychiatry. Res Publ Assoc Res Nerv Ment Dis, 47.* Baltimore, Williams & Wilkins.

176. Gurin, G., Verhoff, J. and Feld, S. (1960): *Americans View their Mental Health. Joint Committee on Mental Illness and Health Monograph No. 4.* New York, Basic Books.

177. Hagnell, O. (1966): *A Prospective Study of the Incidence of Mental*

Disorder. Scandinavian University Books. Stockholm, Norstedts-Bonniers.

178. Hailey, A. M. (1971): Long-stay psychiatric in-patients: a study based on the Camberwell Register. *Psychol Med, 1,* 128.

179. Hamer, Sir W.H. (1928): *Epidemiology Old and New*. London, Kegan Paul, Trench, Trubner & Co. Ltd.

180. Hamman, L. (1939): The relationships of psychiatry to internal medicine. *Ment Hyg, 23:* 177.

181. Hare, E.H. (1955): Mental illness and social class in Bristol. *Br J Prev Soc Med, 9:* 191.

182. Hare, E.H. (1956): Mental illness and social conditions in Bristol. *J Ment Sci, 102:* 349.

183. Hare, E.H. (1956): Family setting and the urban distribution of schizophrenia. *J Ment Sci, 102:* 753.

184. Hare, E.H. and Shaw, G.K. (1965) : *Mental Health on a New Housing Estate: a comparative study of health in two districts of Croydon*. Maudsley Monograph No. 12. London, Oxford University Press.

185. Hare, E.H. and Wing, J.K. (1970): *Psychiatric Epidemiology*. London, Oxford University Press for the Nuffield Prov. Hosp. Trust.

186. Harvey-Smith, E.A. and Cooper, B. (1970): Patterns of neurotic illness in the community. *J Roy Coll Gen Practit, 19:* 132.

187. Hathaway, S.R. and Meehl, P.E. (1951): *An Atlas for the Minnesota Multiphasic Personality Inventory*. London, Oxford University Press.

188. Hawker, A., Edwards, G. and Hensman, C. (1967): Problem drinkers on the pay-roll: an enquiry in one London borough. *Medical Officer, 117:* 313.

189. Hawkins, J. and Williams, D. (1963): Total abdominal hysterectomy. 1,000 consecutive unselected operations. *J Obstet Gynaecol Br Commonw, 70:* 20.

190. Hecker, J.F.C. (1859): *The Epidemics of the Middle Ages*, 3rd ed. Trans. Babington, B.G. New York and London, Trubner.

191. Helgason, T. (1964): Epidemiology of mental disorders in Iceland. *Acta Psychiatr Scand, 40 (Suppl. 173)*.

192. Hempel, C.G. (1961): Introduction to problems of taxonomy. In Zubin, J, (Ed.): *Field Studies in the Mental Disorders*. New York and London, Grune & Stratton.

193. Henderson, J.G., Strachan, R.W., Beck, J.S., Dawson, A. and Daniels, M. (1966): The antigastric-antibody test as a screening procedure for vitamin B_{12} deficiency in psychiatric practice. *Lancet, 2:* 809.

194. Herbert, V. (1964): Studies of folate deficiency in man. *Proc Roy Soc Med, 57:* 377.

195. Heston, L.L. (1966): Psychiatric disorders in foster home reared children of schizophrenic mothers. *Br. J. Psychiatry, 112:* 819.

196. Hewitt, L.E. and Jenkins, R.L. (1946): *The Fundamental Patterns of Maladjustment.* Springfield, Thomas.
197. Hilgard, J.B. and Newman, M.F. (1963): Early parental deprivation in schizophrenia and alcoholism. *Am J Orthopsychiatry, 33:* 409.
198. Hill, Sir A.B. (1955): Snow—an appreciation. *Proc Roy Soc Med, 48:* 1008.
199. Hill, D. and Pond, D.A. (1952): Reflections on one hundred capital cases submitted to electroencephalography. *J Ment Sci, 98:* 23.
200. Hill, O.W. and Price, J.S. (1967): Childhood bereavement and adult depression. *Br J Psychiatry, 113:* 743.
201. Himmelweit, H.T., Oppenheim, A.N. and Vince, P. (1958): *Television and the Child.* London, Oxford University Press for the Nuffield Foundation.
202. Hinckle, L.E. and Wolff, H.C. (1957): The nature of man's adaptation to his total environment and the relation of this to illness. *Arch Intern Med, 99:* 442.
203. Holland, W.W., Doll, R. and Carter, C.O. (1962): Mortality from leukaemia and other cancers among patients with Down's syndrome (mongols) and among their parents. *Br J Cancer, 16:* 177.
204. Hollingshead, A.B. and Redlich, F.C. (1958): *Social Class and Mental Illness.* New York, Wiley.
205. Holmboe, R. and Astrup, C. (1957): A follow-up study of 255 patients with acute schizophrenia and schizophreniform psychoses. *Acta Psychiatr Scand, 32* (Suppl. 115).
206. Holst, Professor (Trans. Massey, A.S.O.) (1852): On the statistics of the insane, blind, deaf and dumb, and lepers, of Norway. *J Stat Soc London, 15:* 250.
207. Hughes, J.N.P. (1966): Alcoholism in Cardiff. *Med Off, 115:* 161.
208. Hunt, R.C., Gruenberg, E.M., Hacken, E. and Huxley, M. (1961): A comprehensive hospital-community service in a state hospital. *Am J Psychiatry, 117:* 817.
209. Hunter, R., Jones, M., Jones, T.G. and Matthews, D.M. (1967): Serum B_{12} and folate concentration in mental patients. *Br J Psychiatry, 113:* 1291.
210. Huntington, G. (1872): On Chorea. *Medical Surgical Reports, 26:* 317.
211. Ibrahim, M., Jenkins, C. Cassel, J., McDonough, J. & Holmes, C. (1966): Personality traits and coronary heart disease. *J Chronic Dis, 19:* 255.
212. Ingham, J.G. (1965): A method for observing symptoms and attitudes. *Br J Clin Soc Psychol, 4:* 131.
213. Jackson, D.D. (Ed.) (1960): *The Aetiology of Schizophrenia.* New York, Basic Books.
214. Jackson, E.W., Turner, J.H., Klauber, M.R. and Norris, F.D. (1968): Down's syndrome: variation of leukaemia occurrence in institutionalized populations. *J Chron Dis, 21:* 247.

215. Jahoda, M. (1958) : *Current Concepts of Positive Mental Health. U.S. Joint Commission on Mental Illness and Health, Monograph Series No. 1.* New York, Basic Books.

216. James, I.P. (1967): Suicide and mortality among heroin addicts in Britain. *Br J Addiction, 62:* 391.

217. Jaspers, K. (1962): *General Psychopathology,* 7th Ed. Trans. Hoenig, J. and Hamilton, M.W. Manchester, Manchester University Press, pp. 383-393.

218. Jellinek, E.M. (1960): *The Disease Concept of Alcoholism.* New Haven, Connecticut, Hillhouse Press.

219. Jenkins, C.D., Rosenman, R.H. and Friedman, M. (1968): Replicability of rating the coronary-prone behavior pattern. *Br J Prev Soc Med, 22:* 16.

220. Jost, H. (1896): Quoted in Diem, O. (1905). Die psychoneurotische erbliche, belastung der geistegesunden und geistekranken. *Arch Rassenbiol, 2:* 215.

221. Kallman, F.J. (1946): The genetic theory of schizophrenia. An analysis of 794 twin index families. *Am J Psychiatry, 103:* 309.

222. Kanner, L. (1957): *Child Psychiatry,* 3rd ed. Springfield, Thomas.

223. Kasl, S.V. and Cobb, S. (1966): Health behaviour, illness behaviour and sick role behaviour. *Arch. Environ Health, 12:* 246.

224. Kawi, A. and Pasamanick, B. (1958): The association of factors of pregnancy with the development of reading disorders in childhood. *JAMA, 166:* 1420.

225. Kay, K.D.W., Beamish, P. and Roth, M. (1964): Old age mental disorders in Newcastle-upon-Tyne. Pt. I. *Br J Psychiatry, 110:* 146.

226. Kay, D.W.K. and Roth, M. (1961): Environmental and hereditary factors in the schizophrenias of old age ('late paraphrenia') and their bearing on the general problem of causation in schizophrenia. *J Ment Sci, 107:* 649.

227. Keith, R.A., Loun, B. and Stare, F.J. (1965): Coronary heart disease and behaviour patterns. *Psychosom Med, 27:* 424.

228. Keller, M. and Efron, V. (1955): The prevalence of alcoholism. *Q J Stud Alcohol, 16:* 619.

229. Kellner, R. (1963) : *Family Ill-health: an investigation in general practice.* London, Tavistock.

230. Kellner, R. and Sheffield, B.F. (1967): Symptom rating test scores in neurotics and normals. *Br J Psychiatry, 113:* 525.

231. Kelly, D.H.W. and Walter, C.J.S. (1968): The relationship between clinical diagnosis and anxiety, assessed by forearm blood flow and other measurements. *Br J Psychiatry, 114:* 611.

232. Kendall, D.G. (1965): Mathematical models of the spread of infection In *Mathematics and Computer Science in Biology and Medicine.* London, H.M.S.O., p. 213.

233. Kendall, M.G. and Babbington Smith, B. (1961): *Tables of Random Sampling Numbers,* 2nd series, impression 4. Cambridge, Cambridge University Press.

234. Kendell, R.E. (1968): *The Classification of Depressive Illness. Maudsley Monograph No. 18.* London, Oxford University Press.

235. Kendell, R.E., Everitt, B., Cooper, J.E., Sartorius, N. and David, M.E. (1968): The reliability of the Present State Examination. *Soc Psychiatry, 3:* 123.

236. Kessel, N. (1960): Psychiatric morbidity in a London general practice. *Br J Prev Soc Med, 14:* 16.

237. Kessel, N. (1965): Self poisoning. *Br Med J, 1:* 1265, 1336.

238. Kessel, N. and Granville-Grossman, K.L. (1961): Suicide in alcoholics. *Br Med J, 2:* 1671.

239. Kessel, N. and Shepherd, M. (1962): Neurosis in hospital and general practice. *J Ment Sci, 108,* 159.

240. Kessel, N. and Shepherd, M. (1965): The health and attitudes of people who seldom consult a doctor. *Med Care (London), 3,* 6.

241. Kety, S.S., Rosenthal, D. Wender, P. and Schulsinger, F. (1968): The types and prevalence of mental illness in the biological and adoptive families of adopted schizophrenics. In Rosenthal, D. and Kety, S.S. (Eds.): *The Transmission of Schizophrenia.* Proc. 2nd Research Conference Foundations' Fund for Research in Psychiatry, Puerto Rico, 1967. Oxford and London, Pergamon Press.

242. Kinsey, A.C., Pomeroy, W.B. and Martin, C.E. (1948): *Sexual Behaviour in the Human Male.* Philadelphia, Saunders.

243. Kinsey, A.C., Pomeroy, W.B., Martin, C.E. and Cebhart, P.H. (1953): *Sexual Behaviour in the Human Female.* Philadelphia, Saunders.

244. Klemperer, J. (1933): Zur belastungsstatistik der durchschnittsbevolkerung. Psychosenhaufigkeit unter 1,000 stickprobenmassig ausgelesenen probanden. *Z Ges Neurol Psychiat, 146:* 277.

245. Knobloch, H. and Pasamanick, B. (1960): Environmental factors affecting human development, before and after birth. *Pediatrics, 26:* 210.

246. Knobloch, H., Rider, R., Harper, P. and Pasamanick, B. (1956): Neuropsychiatric sequelae of prematurity: a longitudinal study. *JAMA, 161:* 581.

247. Knox, S.J. (1961): Severe psychiatric disturbance in the post-operative period: a 5-year survey of Belfast hospitals. *J Ment Sci, 107:* 1078.

248. Kogon, A., Kronmal, R. and Peterson, D.R. (1968): The relationship between infectious hepatitis and Down's syndrome. *Am J Publ Health, 58:* 305.

249. Kraepelin, E. (1909) : *Psychiatrie,* 8th ed. Leipzig, Thieme, vol. 1.

250. Kramer, M. (1961) : Genetical etiology in mental illness: discussion. In: *Causes of Mental Disorder: a review of epidemiological knowledge.* 1959. New York, Milbank Mem. Fund.

251. Kreitman, N. (1961): The reliability of psychiatric diagnosis. *J Ment Sci, 107:* 876.
252. Kreitman, N. (1964): The patient's spouse. *Br J Psychiatry, 110:* 159.
253. Kreitman, N., Collins, J., Nelson, B. and Troop, J. (1970): Neurosis and marital interaction: I. personality and symptoms. *Br J Psychiatry, 117:* 33.
254. Kreitman, N., Smith, P. and Tan, E. (1969): Attempted suicide in social networks. *Br J Prev Soc Med, 23:* 116.
255. Kringlen, E. (1966): Schizophrenia in twins. *Psychiatry, 29:* 172.
256. Krivit, W. and Good, R.A. (1956): The simultaneous occurrence of leukaemia and mongolism: report of 4 cases. *Am J Dis Child, 91:* 218.
257. Kushlick, A. (1966): A community service for the mentally subnormal. *Soc Psychiatry, 1:* 73.
258. Kushlick, A. (1969): A method of evaluating the effectiveness of a community health service. New York, U.N. Study Group on Meaning and Implications of Community Care.
259. Lader, M.H. and Wing, L. (1966): *Physiological Measures, Sedative Drugs and Morbid Anxiety. Maudsley Monograph No. 14.* London, Oxford University Press.
260. A new clinical entity? Leading article, *Lancet, 1:* 789, 1956.
261. Mental symptoms in vitamin B_{12} deficiency. Leading article, *Lancet, 2:* 628, 1965.
262. The pink spot: a red herring? Annotation. *Lancet, 2:* 849, 1966.
263. Landis, C. and Page, J.D. (1938): *Modern Society and Mental Disease.* New York, Farrar & Rhinehart.
264. Langfeldt, G. (1937): The prognosis in schizophrenia and the factors influencing the course of the disease. *Acta Psychiatr Neurol Scand,* Suppl. 13.
265. Lapouse, R. (1967): Problems in studying the prevalence of psychiatric disorder. *Am J Publ Health, 57:* 947.
266. Lapouse, R., Monk, M.A. and Street, E. (1964): A method for use in epidemiological studies of behaviour disorders in children. *Am J Publ Health, 54:* 207.
267. Larsson, L.E., Melin, K.A., Nordström-Öhrberg, G., Silverskiöld, B.P. and Öhrberg, K. (1954): Acute head injuries in boxers: clinical and electro-encephalographic studies. *Acta Psychiatr Neurol Scand,* Suppl. 95.
268. Larsson, T. and Sjögren, T. (1954): A methodological, psychiatric and statistical study of a large Swedish rural population. *Acta Psychiatr Neurol Scand, (Suppl. 89).*
269. Leighton, D.C., Harding, J.S., Macklin, D.B., Macmillan, A.M. and Leighton, A.H. (1963): *The Character of Danger. Psychiatric Symptoms in Selected Communities. The Stirling County Study of Psychi-*

atric *Disorder and Sociocultural Environment*. New York, Basic Books, vol. III.

270. Lemkau, P.V. (1955): The epidemiological study of mental illnesses and mental health. *Am J Psychiatry, 111:* 801.

271. Lemkau, P., Tietze, E. and Cooper, M. (1941): Mental hygiene problems in an urban district. *Ment Hyg, 25:* 624; *26:* 100 & 275; *27:* 279.

272. Lennox, W.G., Gibbs, E.L. and Gibbs, F.A. (1940): Inheritance of cerebral dysrhythmia and epilepsy. *Arch Neurol Psychiatr, 44:* 1155.

273. Lewis, A.J. (1953): Health as a social concept. *Br J Sociol, 4:* 109.

274. Lewis, A.J. (1955): The relation between operative risk and the patients' general condition. Report of the sixteenth "Congress Internationel de Chirurgie," Copenhagen.

275. Lewis, A.J. (1967): Empirical or rational?: The nature and basis of psychiatry. *Lancet, 2:* 1.

276. Lewis, B.I. (1952): Psychosomatic disorders and the non-psychiatrist. *JAMA, 150:* 776.

277. Lewis, B.I. (1953): Psychomedical survey of a private out-patient clinic in a university hospital. *Am J Med, 14:* 586.

278. Lewis, E.O. (1929): *Report on an investigation into the incidence of mental deficiency in six areas, 1925-1927. Report of the Mental Deficiency Committee of the Board of Education and Board of Control, Part IV*. London: H.M.S.O.

279. Lewis, H. (1954): *Deprived Children*. London, Oxford University Press for the Nuffield Foundation.

280. Lilienfeld, A.M. (1957): Epidemiological methods and influences in studies of non-infectious diseases. *Public Health Rep, 72:* 51.

281. Lilienfeld, A. and Pasamanick, B. (1954): Association of maternal and foetal factors with the development of epilepsy. I. Abnormalities in the prenatal and paranatal periods. *JAMA, 155:* 719.

282. Lilienfeld, A. and Pasamanick, B. (1955): The association of prenatal and paranatal factors with the development of cerebral palsy and epilepsy. *Am J Obstet Gynaecol, 70:* 93.

283. Lin, T-Y (1953): A study of the incidence of mental disorder in Chinese and other cultures. *Psychiatry, 16:* 313.

284. Lin, T-Y and Standley, C.C. (1962): *The Scope of Epidemiology in Psychiatry. Public Health Papers, No. 16*. Geneva, W.H.O.

285. Little, J.C. and Kerr, T.A. (1968): Some differences between published norms and data from matched controls as a basis for comparison with psychologically-disturbed groups. *Br J Psychiatry, 114:* 883.

286. Logan, W.P.D. and Brooke, E.M. (1957): *The Survey of Sickness, 1943-1952. Studies on Medical and Population Subjects, No. 12*. London, H.M.S.O.

287. Lotter, V. (1967): Epidemiology of autistic conditions in young children.

Pt. II: some characteristics of the parents and children. *Soc Psychiatry, 1:* 163.

288. Luxenberger, H. (1928): Demographische und psychiatrische Untersuchungen in der engeren biologischen Familie von Paralytikerehegatten. *Z Neurol, 112:* 331.

289. Luxenberger, H. (1928): Vorläufiger bericht über psychiatrischen serieuntersuchungen an zwillingen. *Z ges Neurol Psychiat, 176:* 297.

290. Lyons, H.A. (1971): Psychiatric sequelae of the Belfast riots. *Br J Psychiatry, 118:* 265.

291. MacDermott, W.R. (1908): The topographical distribution of insanity. *Br. Med J, 2:* 950.

292. MacDonald, G., Cuellar, C.B. and Fall, C.V. (1968): The dynamics of malaria. *Bull WHO, 38:* 743.

293. MacFarlane, J.W., Allen, L. and Honzik, M.P. (1954): *A Developmental Study of the Behaviour Problems of Normal Children between 21 Months and 14 Years.* Berkeley & Los Angeles, University of California Press.

294. MacLean, N., Harnden, D.G., Court Brown, W.M., Bond, J. and Mantle, D.J. (1964) : Sex chromosome abnormalities in newborn babies, *Lancet, 1:* 286.

295. MacMahon, B. and Sawa, J.M. (1961): Physical damage to the foetus In: *Causes of Mental Disorders: a review of epidemiological knowledge, 1959.* New York, Milbank Memorial Fund.

296. MacMillan, A.M. (1959): A survey technique for estimating the prevalence of psychoneurotic and related types of disorder in communities. In *Epidemiology of Mental Disorder.* Pasamanick B. (Ed.) New York, Amer. Assoc. for Advancement of Science, Publication No. 60, p. 203.

297. MacMillan, D. (1957): Hospital-community relationships. In *Proc. of 34th Annual Conference of the Milbank Memorial Fund.* New York.

298. MacMillan, D. (1958): Mental health services of Nottingham. *Int J Soc Psychiatry, 4:* 5.

299. MacMillan, D. and Shaw, P. (1966): Senile breakdown in standards of personal and environmental cleanliness. *Br Med J, 2:* 1032.

300. Mai, F.M.M. (1968): Personality and stress in coronary disease. *J Psychosom Res, 12,* 275.

301. Main, T.F. (1946) : Forward psychiatry in the Army: discussion *Proc Roy Soc Med, 39:* 137.

302. Malmo, R.B. and Shagass, C. (1949): Physiologic study of symptom mechanisms in psychiatric patients under stress. *Psychosom Med, 11:* 25.

303. Malzberg, B. (1940): *Social and Biological Aspects of Mental Disease.* Utica, New York, State Press.

304. Malzberg, B. (1955): Mental diseases amongst the native and foreign born white population of New York State. *Ment Hyg, 39:* 545.

305. Malzberg, B. and Lee, E.S. (1956): *Migration and Mental Disease: A study of first admissions to hospitals for mental disease,* New York, 1939-1941. New York, Social Science Research Council.

306. Mannheim, H. and Wilkins, L.T. (1955): *Prediction Methods in Relation to Borstal Training.* London, H.M.S.O.

307. Marinker, M.L. (1969): The general practitioner as family doctor. *J Roy Coll Gen Practit, 17:* 227.

308. Marshall, A.N. and Goldhammer, H. (1955): An application of Markov processes to the study of the epidemiology of mental disease. *J A Statist Assoc, 50:* 99.

309. Massey, F.J. (1970): Computers in epidemiology. In Holland, W.W. (Ed.): *Data Handling in Epidemiology.* London, Oxford University Press.

310. Maudsley, H. (1872): Is insanity on the increase? *Br Med J, 1:* 36.

311. Maxwell, A.E. (1970): Multivariate analysis. In Holland, W.W. (Ed): *Data Handling in Epidemiology.* London, Oxford University Press.

312. Maxwell, A.E. (1971): Agreement among raters. *Br J Psychiatry, 118:* 659.

313. Mayer-Gross, W. (1948): Mental health survey in a rural area. *Eugen Rev, 40:* 140.

314. Mazer, M. (1966): A psychiatric and parapsychiatric register for an island community. *Arch Gen Psychiatry, 14:* 366.

315. McCord, W. and McCord, J. (1959): *Origins of Crime.* New York, Columbia University Press.

316. McEvedy, C.P. and Beard, A.W. (1970): Royal Free epidemic of 1955: a reconsideration. *Br Med J, 1:* 7.

317. McEvedy, C.P. and Beard, A.W. (1970): Concept of benign myalgic encephalomyelitis. *Br Med J, 1:* 11.

318. McEvedy, C.P., Griffith, A. and Hall, T. (1966): Two school epidemics. *Br Med J, 2:* 1300.

319. McLean, F. (1932): Psychiatry and general medicine. *Ment Hyg (New York), 16:* 577.

320. Mechanic, D. (1962): Some factors in identifying and defining mental illness. *Ment Hyg: 46,* 66.

321. Mechanic, D. (1970): Problems and prospects in psychiatric epidemiology In Hare, E.H. and Wing, J.K. (Eds.): *Psychiatric Epidemiology.* London, Oxford University Press for the Nuffield Provincial Hospitals Trust.

322. Medical Research Council (1963): Treatment of phenylketonuria: report to the M.R.C. of the conference on phenylketonuria. *Br Med J, 1:* 1691.

323. Metrakos, J.D. (1963): The centrencephalic E.E.G. in epilepsy. *Proc 2nd Int Congr Hum Genet, 3:* 1792, 1961, Rome.
324. Meyer, A. (1951). Winters, E.E. (Ed.): *Collected Papers. Vol. III.* Baltimore: Johns Hopkins Press.
325. Meyer, R.J. and Haggerty, R.J. (1962): Streptococcal infections in families. *Pediatrics, 29:* 539.
326. Mezey, A.G. (1960): Personal background, emigration and mental disorder in Hungarian refugees. *J Ment Sci, 106:* 618.
327. Milbank Memorial Fund (1950): *Epidemiology of Mental Disorder.* New York.
328. Ministry of Health (1962): *National Health Service: A Hospital Plan for England and Wales.* London, H.M.S.O., Cmnd. 1604.
329. Moersch, F.P. (1932): Psychiatry in medicine. *Am J Psychiatry, 11:* 831.
330. Monck, E.M. (1963): Employment experiences in 127 discharged schizophrenic men in London. *Br J Prev Soc Med, 17:* 101.
331. Morris, J.N. (1957): *Uses of Epidemiology.* Edinburgh, Livingstone.
332. Moser, C.A. and Kalton, G. (1971): *Survey Methods in Social Investigation.* 2nd ed. London, Heinemann.
333. Moser, C. and Scott, W. (1961): *British Towns.* Edinburgh, Oliver & Boyd.
334. Moss, M.C. and Beresford Davies, E. (1967): *A Survey of Alcoholism in an English County.* Altrincham, Cheshire, St. Ann's Press, for Geigy.
335. Moss, P.D. and McEvedy, C.P. (1966): An epidemic of overbreathing among schoolgirls. *Br Med J, 2:* 1295.
336. Motto, J.A. (1970) : Newspaper influence on suicide: a controlled study. *Arch Gen Psychiatry, 23:* 143.
337. Muhsam, H.V. (1970): Models for infectious diseases. In Holland, W.W. (Ed.): *Data Handling in Epidemiology.* London, Oxford University Press.
338. Murphy, H.B.M. (1961): Social change and mental health. In *Causes of Mental Disorder: a review of epidemiological knowledge, 1959.* New York, Milbank Memorial Fund.
339. Murphy, H.B. and Raman, A.C. (1971): The chronicity of schizophrenia in indigenous tropical peoples: results of a twelve year follow-up survey. *Br J Psychiatry, 118:* 489.
340. Murphy, H.B., Wittkower, E.D. and Chance, N.A. (1964): Cross-cultural enquiry into the symptomatology of depression. *Transcultural Psychiatric Research Review and Newsletter, 1:* 5.
341. Murphy, H.B., Wittkower, E.D., Fried, J. and Ellenberger, H. (1963): A cross-cultural survey of schizophrenic symptomatology. *Int J Soc Psychiatry, 9:* 237.
342. Naecke, P. (1898): Die Sogenannten äusseren degenerationszeichen bei der progressiven paralyse u.s.w. *Allg z Psychiat, 55:* 557.

343. Navarro, V. (1969): Systems approach to health planning. *Health Serv Res, 4:* 96.

344. Nelson, B., Collins, J., Kreitman, N. and Troop, J. (1970): Neurosis and marital interaction. II. Time sharing and social activity. *Br J Psychiatry, 117:* 47.

345. New York State Department of Mental Hygiene (1959): A mental health survey of older people. *Psychiatr Q, (special supplement):* 45, 252.

346. Nielsen. J., Suboi, T.T., Sturup, G. and Romano, D. (1968): XYY chromosomal constitution in criminal psychopaths. *Lancet, 2:* 576.

347. Norris, V. (1959): *Mental Illness in London. Maudsley Monograph, No. 6.* London, Chapman & Hall.

348. O'Connor, N. (1958): The prevalence of mental defect. In Clarke, A.D.B. and Clarke, A.M. (Eds.): *Mental Deficiency: The Changing Outlook,* London, Methuen.

349. Ødegaard, Ø. (1932): Emigration and insanity. *Acta Psychiatr Scand, (Suppl. 4).*

350. Ødegaard, Ø. (1952): The incidence of mental diseases as measured by census investigation versus admission statistics. *Psychiatr Q, 26:* 212.

351. Ødegaard, Ø. (1956): The incidence of psychosis in various occupations. *Int J Soc Psychiatr, 2:* 85.

352. Ødegaard, Ø. (1961): The epidemiology of depressive psychoses *in* 'Depression.' *Acta Psychiatr Scand, 37 (Suppl. 162).*

353. Ødegaard, Ø. (1967): Changes in the prognosis of the functional psychoses since the days of Kraepelin. *Br J Psychiatry, 113:* 813.

354. Oltman, J.E. and Friedman, S. (1965): Report on parental deprivation in psychiatric disorders. I. In schizophrenia. *Arch Gen Psychiatr, 12:* 46.

355. Opler, M.K. (1956): *Culture, Psychiatry and Human Values.* Springfield, Illinois, Thomas.

356. Ostfeld, A.M., Lebovits, B., Shekelle, R.B. and Paul, O. (1964): A prospective study of the relationship between personality and coronary heart disease. *J Chron Dis, 17:* 265.

357. Paffenbarger, R.S. (1964): Epidemiological aspects of post-partum mental illness. *Br J Prev Soc Med, 18:* 189.

358. Paffenbarger, R.S. and Asnes, D.P. (1966): Chronic disease in former college students. III. Precursors of suicide in early and middle life. *Am J Publ Health, 56:* 1026.

359. Parloff, M.B., Kellman, H.C. and Frank, J.D. (1954): Comfort, effectiveness and self-awareness as criteria of improvement in psychotherapy. *Am J Psychiatr 111:* 343.

360. Pasamanick, B. (1961): Epidemiological investigations of some prenatal factors in the production of neuropsychiatric disorders. In Hoch, P.H. and Zubin, J. (Eds.): *Comparative Epidemiology of the Mental Disorders.* New York & London, Grune & Stratton, p. 260.

361. Pasamanick, B., Constantinou, F.K. and Lilienfeld, A.M. (1956): Pregnancy experience and the development of childhood speech disorder: an epidemiological study of the association with maternal and foetal factors. *AMA J Dis Child, 91:* 113.

362. Pasamanick, B. and Kawi, A. (1956): A study of the association of prenatal and paranatal factors with the development of tics in children: a preliminary investigation. *J Pediatr, 48:* 596.

363. Pasamanick, B., Rogers, M.E. and Lilienfeld, A.M. (1956): Pregnancy experience and the development of childhood behaviour disorders. *Am J Psychiatr, 112:* 613.

364. Paul, J.R. (1958): *Clinical Epidemiology.* University of Chicago Press.

365. Payne, L.C. (1966): *An Introduction to Medical Automation.* London, Pitman.

366. Pearson, K. and Jaederholm, G.A. (1931): On the inheritance of mental disease. *Annals of Eugenics (London), 4:* 362.

367. Pearson, R.S.B. (1938): Psychoneurosis in hospital practice. *Lancet, 1;* 451.

368. Peck, P.F. and Havighurst, R.J. (1960): *The Psychology of Character Development.* New York, Wiley.

369. Pedder, J.R. and Goldberg, D.P. (1970): A survey by questionnaire of psychiatric disturbance in patients attending a venereal diseases clinic. *Br J Vener Dis, 46:* 58.

370. Pemberton, J. (1951): A socio-medical study of 200 hospital medical patients. *Lancet, 1:* 224.

371. Penrose, L.S. (1938): *A clinical and genetic study of 1,280 cases of mental defect (Colchester Survey). Special Report Medical Research Council, No. 229.* London, H.M.S.O.

372. Penrose, L.S. (1963): *Biology of Mental Defect,* 2nd ed. New York, Grune & Stratton.

373. Penrose, L.S. (1970): The contribution of cytogenetics to clinical psychology. In Price, J.H. (Ed.): *Modern Trends in Psychological Medicine: 2.* London, Butterworths.

374. Perris, C. (1966): A study of bipolar (manic depressive) and unipolar recurrent depressive psychosis. II. Childhood environment and precipitating factors. *Acta Psychiat Scand, 45(Suppl. 194).*

375. Perry, T.L., Hansen, S., MacDougall, L. and Schwarz, C.J. (1967): Studies of amines in normal and schizophrenic subjects. In Himwich, H.E., Kety, S.S. and Smythies, J.R. (Eds.): *Amines and Schizophrenia.* Oxford & London, Pergamon Press.

376. Perry, T.L., Hansen, S. and MacIntyre, L. (1964): Failure to detect 3-4 dimethyl-phenyl-ethylamine in the urine of schizophrenics. *Nature, 202:*519.

377. Pfister-Ammende, M. (1955): The symptomatology, treatment and prog-

nosis in mentally ill refugees and repatriates in Switzerland. In Murphy, H.B.M. (Ed.): *Flight and Resettlement.* Unesco, Paris.

378. Pickles, W.N. (1939): *Epidemiology in Country Practice.* Bristol, John Wright.

379. Plunkett, R.J. and Gordon, J.E. (1960): *Epidemiology and Mental Illness.* New York, Basic Books.

380. Pond, D.A. and Bidwell, B.H. (1960): A survey of epilepsy in 14 general practices. II. Social and psychological aspects. *Epilepsia, 1:* 285.

381. Post, F. (1962): The social orbit of psychiatric patients. *J Ment Sci, 108:* 759.

382. Prys Williams, G. and Glatt, M.M. (1966) : The incidence of (longstanding) alcoholism in England and Wales. *Br J Addict, 61:* 257.

383. Pugh, T.F., Jerath, B.K., Schmidt, W.M. and Reed, R.B. (1963): Rates of mental diseases related to childbearing. *N Engl J Med, 268:*1224.

384. Rahe, R.H., McKean, J.D. and Arthur, R.J. (1967): A longitudinal study of life-change and illness patterns. *J Psychosom Res, 10:* 355.

385. Rawnsley, K. (1968): Epidemiology of affective disorders. In Coppen, A. and Walk, A. (Eds.): *Recent Developments in Affective Disorders: a Symposium.* Ashford, Kent, Headley Brothers, for R.M.P.A.

386. Rawnsley, K. (1968): Social attitudes and psychiatric epidemiology. In Shepherd, M. and Davies, D.L. (Eds.): *Studies in Psychiatry.* London, Oxford University Press.

387. Ray, Isaac (1873) : *Contributions to Mental Pathology.* Boston, Little, Brown & Co.

388. Registrar General (1954): *Measurement of Morbidity. Report of the statistics sub-committee on medical nomenclature and statistics. General Register Office, Studies of Medical and Population Subjects No. 8.* London, H.M.S.O.

389. Reid, D.D. (1960) : *Epidemiological methods in the study of mental disorders. Public Health Papers No. 2.* Geneva, W.H.O.

390. Rennie, Drummond (1970): After the earthquake. *Lancet, 2:* 704.

391. Rennie, T.A.C. (1942) : Prognosis in manic-depressive psychoses. *Am J Psychiatry, 98:* 801.

392. Reynolds, E.H., Milner, G., Matthews, D.M. and Chanarin, I. (1966): Anticonvulsant therapy, magaloblastic haemopoiesis and folic acid metabolism. *Q J Med, 35:* 521.

393. Reynolds, G.P. (1930): The aetiology of psychoneurosis encountered in the practice of internal medicine. *N Engl J Med, 203:* 312.

394. Roberts, J.A.F. (1948): The frequencies of the ABO blood-groups in South-Western England. *Ann Eugenics, 14:* 109.

395. Robins, L.N. (1966) : *Deviant Children Grown Up: a sociological and psychiatric study of sociopathic personality.* Baltimore, Williams and Wilkins.

396. Robinson, J.O. (1962): A study of neuroticism and casual arterial blood pressure. *Br J Soc Clin Psychol, 2:* 56.

397. Roessler, R. and Greenfield, N.S. (1961): Incidence of somatic disease in psychiatric patients. *Psychosom Med, 23:* 413.

398. Rogers, M.E., Lilienfeld, A.M. and Pasamanick, B. (1955): Prenatal and paranatal factors in the development of childhood behaviour disorders. *Acta Psychiatr Scand, (Suppl. 102).*

399. Rosanoff, A.J. (1917): Survey of mental disorders in Nassau County, New York, July-October 1916. *Psychiatr Bull (Houston), 2:* 109.

400. Rosenman, R.H., Friedman, M., Strauss, R., Wurm, M., Jenkins, C.D. and Messinger, H.B. (1966): Coronary heart disease in the Western Collaborative Group Study. *JAMA, 195:* 86.

401. Rosenthal, D. (1968): The heredity-environment issue in schizophrenia: summary of the conference and present status of our knowledge. In Rosenthal, D. and Kety, S. (Eds.): *The Transmission of Schizophrenia.* Proc. 2nd Conf. Res. Psychiat., Puerto Rico, 1967. Oxford & London, Pergamon Press.

402. Roth, M. (1955): The natural history of mental disorder in old age. *J Ment Sci, 101:* 281.

403. Roth, M. and Morrissey, J.D. (1952): Problems in the diagnosis and classification of mental disorder in old age. *J Ment Sci, 98:* 66.

404. Roth, W.F. and Luton, F.H. (1942): The mental health program in Tennessee. *Amer J Psychiatr, 99:* 662.

405. Rowntree, G. (1955): Early childhood in broken families. *Population Studies, 8:* 247.

406. Royal College of Obstetricians and Gynaecologists and the Population Investigation Committee (1948). *Maternity in Great Britain.* London, Oxford University Press.

407. Rüdin, Ernst (1916): Zur vererbung und neuentstehung der dementia praecox. Berlin, Springer.

408. Rutter, M.L. (1966): *Children of Sick Parents: An Environmental and Psychiatric Study. Maudsley Monograph No. 16.* London, Oxford University Press.

409. Rutter, M.L. (1970). Sex differences in children's responses to family stress. In Anthony, E.J. and Koupernik, C. (Eds.): *International Year Book of Child Psychiatry.* The Child in his Family. New York, Wiley, vol. 1.

410. Rutter, M. and Brown, G.W. (1966): The reliability and validity of measures of family life and relationships in families containing a psychiatric patient. *Soc Psychiatry, 1:* 38.

411. Rutter, M.L., Graham, P. and Whitmore, K. (1970). *Education, Health and Behaviour.* London, Longmans.

412. Rutter, M.L., Graham, P. and Yule, W. (1970). *A Neuropsychiatric*

study in childhood. Spastics International Medical Publications. London, Heinemann. Philadelphia, Lippincott.

413. Rutter, M., Lebovici, S., Eisenberg, L., Snezevskij, A.V., Sadoun, R., Brooke, E. and Lin, T.Y. (1969): A triaxial classification of mental disorders in childhood: an international study. *J Child Psychol Psychiatry, 10:* 41.

414. Ryle, J.A. (1936): *The Natural History of Disease.* London, Oxford University Press.

415. Sainsbury, P. (1960): Neurosis and psychosomatic disorders in out-patients. *Adv Psychosom Med, 1:* 259.

416. Sayed, Z.A., Lewis, S.A. and Brittain, R.P. (1969): An electroencephalographic and psychiatric study of 32 insane murderers. *Br J Psychiatry, 115:* 1115.

417. Schmidt, H.O. and Fonda, C.P. (1956): The reliability of psychiatric diagnosis: a new look. *J Abnorm Soc Psychol, 52:* 262.

418. Scottish Council for Research in Education (1949) : *The Trend of Scottish Intelligence.* London, University of London Press.

419. Seager, C.P. (1960): A controlled study of post partum mental illness. *J Ment Sci, 106:* 214.

420. Shepherd, M. (1957) : *A Study of the Major Psychoses in an English County. Maudsley Monograph No. 3.* London, Chapman & Hall.

421. Shepherd, M., Brooke, E.M., Cooper, J.E. and Lin, T.Y. (1968): An experimental approach to psychiatric diagnosis: an international study. *Acta Psychiatr Scand, 44 (Suppl. 201).*

422. Shepherd, M. and Cooper, B. (1964): Epidemiology and mental disorder: a review. *J Neurol Neurosurg Psychiatr, 27:*277.

423. Shepherd, M., Cooper, B., Brown, A.C. and Kalton, G.W. (1966): *Psychiatric Illness in General Practice.* London, Oxford University Press.

424. Shepherd, M., Goodman, N. and Watt, D.C. (1961): The application of hospital statistics in the evaluation of pharmacotherapy in a psychiatric population. *Comp Psychiatry, 2:* 11.

425. Shepherd, M., Oppenheim, A.N. and Mitchell, S. (1971): *Childhood Behaviour and Mental Health.* London, University of London Press.

426. Shields, J. (1967): The genetics of schizophrenia in historical context. In Coppen, A. and Walk, A. (Eds.): *Recent Developments in Schizophrenia: a Symposium.* Ashford, Kent, Headley Brothers for R.M.P.A.

427. Shields, J. and Slater, E. (1967): Genetic aspects of schizophrenia. *Hospital Medicine (London), 1:* 579.

428. Shulman, R. (1967): A survey of vitamin B_{12} deficiency in an elderly psychiatric population. *Br J Psychiatr, 113:* 241.

429. Siler, J.F., Garrison, P.E. and MacNeal, W.L. (1914): Pellagra: a sum-

mary of the first progress report of the Thompson-McFadden Pellagra Commission. *JAMA, 62:* 8.

430. Siler, J.F., Garrison, P.E. and MacNeal, W.L. (1914): Further studies of the Thompson-McFadden Pellagra Commission. A summary of the second progress report. *JAMA, 63:* 1090.

431. Slater, E. (1958): The monogenic theory of schizophrenia. *Acta Genet (Basel), 8:* 50.

432. Slater, E. and Woodside, M. (1951): *Patterns of Marriage. A study of marriage relationships in the urban working classes.* London, Cassell.

433. Sloane, R., Habit, A., Eveson, M. and Payne, R. (1961): Some behavioural and other correlates of cholesterol metabolism. *J Psychosom Res, 5:* 183.

434. Smith, G.F. (1970): The investigation of the mental effects of trichlorethylene. *Ergonomics, 13,* 580.

435. Sokal, R.R. and Sneath, P.H.A. (1963): *Principles of Numerical Taxonomy.* San Francisco & London, Freeman.

436. Spitzer, R.L. and Endicott, J. (1967): Diagno: a computer program for psychiatric diagnosis utilizing the differential diagnosis procedure. *Arch Gen Psychiat, 183,* 746.

437. Spitzer, R.L., Endicott, J. and Fliess, J.L. (1967): Instruments and recording forms for evaluating psychiatric status and history. Rationale, method of development and description. *Compr Psychiatry, 8:* 321.

438. Spitzer, R.L., Fliess, J.L., Burdock, E. and Hardesty, A. (1964): The mental status schedule: rationale, reliability and validity. *Compr Psychiatry, 5:* 384.

439. Srole, L., Langner, T.S., Michael, S.T., Opler, M.K.N. and Rennie, T.A.C. (1962): *Mental Health in the Metropolis: the Mid-town Manhattan Study.* Vol. 1. New York, McGraw Hill.

440. State of Massachusetts (1855): Report of a commission to examine statistics of lunacy and conditions of asylums in the State of Massachusetts, 1855. Available only in photocopy from National Library, Washington, D.C.

441. Stengel, E. (1967): Recent developments in classification. In Coppen, A. and Walk, A. (Eds.): *Recent Developments in Schizophrenia: a Symposium.* Ashford, Kent, Headley Brothers for R.M.P.A.

442. Stenstedt, A. (1952): A study in manic-depressive psychoses: clinical social and genetic investigation. *Acta Psychiatr Neurol Scand,* (Suppl. 29).

443. Stenstedt, A. (1959): Involutional melancholia: an aetiological, clinical, and social study of endogenous depression in later life with special reference to genetic factors. *Acta Psychiatr Scand,* (Suppl. 127).

444. Stoller, A. and Collman, R.D. (1965): Incidence of infective hepatitis followed by Down's syndrome 9 months later. *Lancet, 2:* 1221.

445. Strauss, H., Rahm, W.E. and Barrera, S.E. (1939): E.E.G. studies in relatives of epileptics. *Proc Soc Exp Biol (N.Y.), 42:* 207.

446. Strömgren, E. (1938): Beiträge zur psychiatrischen erblehre. *Acta Psychiatr Scand, (Suppl. 19).*

447. Strömgren, E. (1950): Statistical and genetical population studies within psychiatry: methods and principal results. *Proc 1st Internat. Congress of Psychiatry, Paris, 1950.* Paris, Herman et cie, Vol. VI, p. 155-192.

448. Temoche, A., Pugh, H.F. and MacMahon, B. (1964): Suicide rates among current and former mental institution patients. *J Neur Ment Dis, 138:* 124.

449. Terris, M. (1962): The scope and methods of epidemiology. *Am J Public Health, 52:* 1371.

450. Terris, M. (Ed.) (1964): *Goldberger on pellagra.* Baton Rouge, Louisiana State University Press.

451. Terris, M. (1965): Use of hospital admissions in epidemiological studies of mental disease. *Arch Gen Psychiatry, 12:* 420.

452. Thurnam, John (1845): *Observations and Essays on the Statistics of Insanity.* London, Simpkin, Marshall.

453. Tienaari, P. (1963): Psychiatric illnesses in identical twins. *Acta Psychiatr Scand, (Suppl. 171).*

454. Tizard, J. (1964): *Community Services for the Mentally Handicapped.* London, Oxford University Press.

455. Tooth, G.C. and Brooke, E.M. (1961): Trends in the mental hospital population. *Lancet, 1:* 710.

456. Truett, J., Cornfield, J. and Kannel, W. (1967): A multivariate analysis of the risk of coronary heart disease in Framingham. *J Chron Dis, 20:* 511.

457. Trussell, R.E. and Elinson, J. (1959): *Chronic illness in a rural area— the Hunterdom Study. Chronic Illness in the United States. Vol. III.* Cambridge, Mass, Commission on Chronic Illness.

458. Tuckman, J. and Youngman, W.F. (1963): Suicide risk among persons attempting suicide. *Public Health Rep, 78:* 585.

459. Tuke, Daniel Hack (1878): *Insanity in Ancient and Modern Life, With Chapter on Its Prevention.* London, MacMillan.

460. Turton, E.C. and Warren, P.K.G. (1960): Dementia: a clinical and E.E.G. study. *J Ment Sci, 106:* 1493.

461. Waisman, H.A. and Gerritsen, T. (1964): Biochemical and clinical correlations. In Stevens, H.A. and Heber, R. (Eds.): *Mental Retardadation: a review of research.* Chicago, University of Chicago Press.

462. Walk, D. (1967): Suicide and community care. *Br J Psychiatry, 113:* 1381.
463. Weinberg, A.A. (1961): *Migration and Belonging.* The Hague, Internat Publications Service.
464. Wender, P.H., Rosenthal, D. and Kety, S. (1968): A psychiatric assessment of the adoptive parents of schizophrenics. In Rosenthal, D. and Kety, S.S. (Eds.): *The Transmission of Schizophrenia.* Oxford and London, Pergamon Press, p. 235-251.
465. West, D.J. (1967): *The Young Offender.* London, Duckworth.
466. West, D.J. (1969): *Present Conduct and Future Delinquency.* London, Heinemann's Educational Books.
467. White, W.A. (1903): The geographical distribution of insanity in the United States. *J Nerv Ment Dis, 30:* 257.
468. Wiener, J.M., Delano, J.G. and Klass, D.W. (1966): An E.E.G. study of delinquent and non-delinquent adolescents. *Arch Gen Psychiatry, 15:* 144.
469. Williams, D. (1969): Neural factors related to habitual aggression. *Brain, 92:* 503.
470. Wilson, C.W.M., Banks, J.A., Mapes, R.E.A. and Korte, S.M.T. (1963): Patterns of prescribing in general practice. *Br Med J, 2:* 604.
471. Wing, J.K. (1961): A simple and reliable sub-classification of chronic schizophrenia. *J Ment Sci, 107,* 862.
472. Wing, J.K. (1967): Social treatment, rehabilitation and management. In Coppen, A. and Walk, A. (Eds.): *Recent Developments in Schizophrenia: a Symposium.* Ashford, Kent, Headley Brothers for R.M.P.A.
473. Wing, J.K. (1970): A standard form of psychiatric present state examination. In Hare, E.H. and Wing, J.K. (Eds.): *Psychiatric Epidemiology.* London, Oxford University Press for the Nuffield Provincial Hospitals Trust.
474. Wing, J.K., Birley, J.L.T., Cooper, J.E., Graham, P. and Isaacs, A.D. (1967): Reliability of a procedure for measuring and classifying "Present Psychiatric State." *Br J Psychiatry, 113:* 499.
475. Wing, J.K. and Brown, G.W. (1970): *Institutionalism and Schizophrenia: a comparative study of three mental hospitals, 1960-1968.* Cambridge, University Press.
476. Wing, J.K., Denham, J. and Monro, A.B. (1959): Duration of stay in hospital of patients suffering from schizophrenia. *Br J Prev Soc Med, 13:* 145.
477. Wing, J.K., Wing, L. and Hailey, A. (1970): The use of case registers for evaluating and planning psychiatric services. In Wing, J.K. and Bransby, R. (Eds.): *Psychiatric Case Registers.* London, Dept. Health & Soc. Security, Statistical Report series.
478. Wing, L. (1970): Observations on the psychiatric section of the Inter-

national Classification of Diseases and the British Glossary of Mental Disorders. *Psychol Med, 1:* 79.

479. Wing, L., Wing, J.K., Hailey, A., Bahn, A.K., Smith, H.E. and Baldwin, J.A. (1967): The use of psychiatric services in three urban areas: an international case register study. *Soc Psychiatry, 116:* 423.

480. Winkler, G.E. and Kove, S.S. (1962): The implications of electroencephalographic abnormalities in homicide cases. *J Neuropsychiatry, 3:* 322.

481. Winslow, C.E.A. (1944): *The Conquest of Epidemic Disease.* Princeton, New Jersey, Princeton University Press.

482. Wootton, B. (1959): *Social Science and Social Pathology.* London, Allen & Unwin.

483. World Health Organization (1960): *Epidemiology of Mental Disorders. 8th Report of the Expert Committee on Mental Health. W.H.O. Technical Report Series, No. 185.* Geneva, W.H.O.

484. World Health Organization (1967): *Manual of the International Statistical Classification of Diseases, Injuries and Causes of Death, 8th Revision.* Geneva, W.H.O.

485. Yap, P.M. (1951): Mental diseases peculiar to certain cultures: a survey of comparative psychiatry. *J Ment Sci, 97:* 313.

486. Yates, F. (1960): *Sampling Methods for Censuses and Surveys,* 3rd ed. London, Griffin & Co.

487. Zung, W. (1965): A self-rating depression scale. *Arch Gen Psychiatry, 12:* 63.

488. Zwerling, I., Titchener, J., Gottschalk, L., Levine, M., Culbertson, W., Cohen, S. and Silver, H. (1955): Personality disorder and the relationships of emotion to surgical illness in 200 surgical patients. *Am J Psychiatry, 112:* 270.

INDEX